nutrition
periodization
for
endurance
athletes

Taking Traditional Sports
Nutrition to the Next Level

BOB SEEBOHAR, MS, RD, CSCS

Bull Publishing company
P.O. Box 1377
Boulder, CO 80306
(800)676-2855
www.bullpub.com
ISBN 0-923521-83-6

Manufactured in the United States of America.

Distributed to the trade by:
Publisher's Group West
1700 Fourth Street
Berkeley, CA 94710

Publisher: James Bull
Project Manager and Manuscript Editor: Erin Mulligan
Cover Design: Lightbourne
Interior Design and Composition: Publication Services, Inc.

Library of Congress Cataloging-in-Publication Data

Seebohar, Bob.
    Nutrition periodization for endurance athletes : taking traditional
sports nutrition to the next level / by Bob Seebohar.
        p. cm.
    Includes index.
    ISBN 0-923521-83-6
    1. Athletes—Nutrition. I. Title.

TX361.A8S44 2004
613.2'024'796—dc22
                            2004013237

10 9 8 7 6 5 4 3 2 1

Dedication

I would like to dedicate this book to endurance sports. Without them, I would not be the athlete, husband, or father that I am and would not have such an appreciation for health, fitness, or life balance.

This journey would not have been possible without the tremendous support of my family. Thank you Wendy, Chase, and Natalie for your unconditional love. And special thanks to my mother who taught me to never give up and to always pursue my dreams no matter what obstacles stood in my way.

The dedication would not be final without my sincere thanks to Ellen Coleman, who has been one of my mentors and who first introduced me to Jim Bull. It was he who adopted my ideas and allowed me to pursue one of my dreams—writing a book.

—Bob Seebohar

Contents

INTRODUCTION   1

1 Periodization 5
What is Periodization? 5
Overtraining and Injury 10

2 Nutrients for Life 15
The Six Essential Nutrients 16
Digestion Basics 17
Carbohydrates 18
Protein 22
Fat 26
Water 32
Vitamins 34
Minerals 38
Fiber 41
Summary 43

3 Nutrition Periodization 47
The Important Role of Nutrition 47
Periodization and Nutrition Planning 49
Macrocycle Nutrition Guidelines 51
Mesocycle and Microcycle Nutrition Guidelines 57
Summary 100

4 Successful Weight Management 101
Making a Lifestyle Change 102
Timing of Weight Loss 102
Basics of Weight Loss 105
Why Fad Diets Don't Work 109
Measure Your RMR 111
Safe Steps to Weight Loss: How to Do It 113
Summary 122

5 Nutrition Supplementation 123

The Nutrition Supplements Market 124
Nutrition Supplements for the Endurance Athlete 130
Summary 146

6 Special Considerations for the Endurance Athlete 149

Dehydration 150
Heat Cramps 154
Hyponatremia 158
Immune System Depression 162
Summary 169

INDEX 171

List of Tables/Figures

LIST OF TABLES

Table 2.1	Composition of Some Oils p. 29
Table 2.2	Approximate EFA Content of Some Popular Oils p. 31
Table 2.3	High-Fiber Favorites p. 44
Table 3.1	Daily Nutrition Needs During the Preparation Mesocycle p. 63
Table 3.2	Training Needs during the Preparation Mesocycle p. 69
Table 3.3	Daily Nutrition Needs during the Pre-race Cycle p. 75
Table 3.4	Training Needs during the Pre-race Cycle p. 76
Table 3.5	Daily Nutrition Needs During the Race Cycle p. 80
Table 3.6	Training Needs during the Race Cycle p. 83
Table 3.7	Daily Nutrition Needs during the Transition Mesocycle p. 97
Table 3.8	Training Needs during the Transition Mesocycle p. 98
Table 6.1	GI and GL Classifications p. 168

LIST OF FIGURES

Figure 1.1	The Periodization Model p. 6
Figure 1.2	Progressive Build and Recovery Weeks of a Mesocycle p. 12
Figure 3.1	Three Cornerstones of Endurance - Training p. 48
Figure 3.2	Nutrition Periodization p. 51
Figure 3.3	Body Weight and Macronutrient Needs pp. 59-61
Figure 4.1	The Energy Balance Equation p. 106
Figure 4.2	Cami's PEBE p. 119

About the Author

Bob Seebohar, MS, RD, CSCS, is a practicing Sports Dietitian who specializes in working with endurance athletes. He has been a competitive endurance athlete since 1993 and has competed in all types and distances of endurance sports, including five Ironman races.

Bob is also a professional endurance coach and owns and operates ATP Coaching (www.atpcoaching.com), which provides professional coaching and sports nutrition services to all ages and abilities of endurance sport athletes.

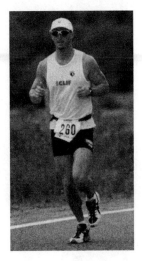

Introduction

A NEW WAY OF THINKING ABOUT NUTRITION

Before you begin reading this book, it is important to understand that you will have to change your way of thinking in order to adopt the principles in it. To get the most out of this book, you will have to relinquish your traditional belief that nutrition is only important a few days or a week prior to, during, and immediately after your event. That is what I call the "old school" way of applying nutrition to training. The "new school" way is to think about nutrition as an important part of your training year-round. Just as you have specific physiological goals for each training cycle (i.e., increasing endurance, strength, and speed), you should have specific nutrition goals as well. Your nutrition plan should support your training, not the other way around.

Think about that for a bit. Your eating program should support your training so that you are able to train efficiently and effectively and improve your health and performance. To elicit

1

positive physiological responses your nutrition must support your body's energy needs as they change with the varying training volume and intensity stressors in your training year. The underlying principle here is that you should eat to train, not train to eat. Before you explore each chapter of this book, make sure that you have a good grasp of what I have just stated. I cannot emphasize enough that you need to be able to think in the "new school" way about nutrition and your yearly training program. This may be a radical departure for you and you may need to re-read chapters in order to leave your "old school" application of sports nutrition behind, but it will be worth it.

Please remember that this is not just another sports nutrition book. The words "sports nutrition" are not in the title for a reason. This book presents concepts and ideas that you have not seen before in other sports nutrition books. For example, in the nutrition supplementation chapter, I do not discuss which supplements are beneficial and which are not. What I do is provide is a full explanation of the ingredients that are found in the nutritional supplements so that you have a good understanding of how they interact with your body. I answer relevant questions such as: Will they cause gastrointestinal distress? Is one product healthier or better for performance than another based on their ingredients? In this book I am giving you information that you haven't heard before, information that you can use to improve your health and performance.

USING THIS BOOK

This book is intended to serve as a workbook that will help you understand how to optimize your nutrition to fit your yearly, monthly, weekly, and daily training and improve your health and performance. Both of these variables—health and performance—are important at all times of the year. Sports nutrition is about improving health *and* performance, not one or the other.

The book begins with a brief explanation of periodization for sport so you understand why you should vary your training throughout the year and what purposes it serves. Then we discuss basics concepts about the six essential nutrients. In Chapter 2, you will find that the nutrition information is presented in a different way from most sports nutrition books. You will then read the most innovative chapter of this book, Chapter 3 on nutrition periodization. The content in this chapter will allow you to structure your daily, weekly, monthly, and yearly nutrition plans based on your current cycle of training. From there, it's on to learning the only tried and true way of weight management and how to manipulate your personal energy balance equation for weight loss, gain, or maintenance. I include the topic of weight control in the book because every endurance athlete will at some point want to manipulate their body weight to affect health and/or performance and I wanted to provide you with the knowledge and skill set to do that safely. Then we cover nutrition supplementation and finally finish with some special considerations that you need to be aware of as an endurance athlete.

ENDURANCE ATHLETES

Who is this book for? Endurance athletes participate in events ranging from 5k's and marathons to the Race Across America (RAAM), Ironman triathlons, and ultra-endurance events such as the Ultraman (6.2-mile swim, 90-mile bike on Day 1, 171.4-mile bike on Day 2, and 52.4-mile run on Day 3), the Sahara Ultra Run (a 3-day, 117.8-mile run across the Sahara Desert), the Manhattan Marathon Swim (a 28.5-mile swim), and the increasingly popular adventure races, which average 1–7 days in length.

It doesn't matter what your choice of sport or distance is. You can be a triathlete, adventure racer, swimmer, cyclist, runner, race walker, or nordic skier. The point is that you enjoy exercise, you believe aerobic exercise is beneficial to your health, and you may want to improve your performance race-to-race or year-to-year. You are an endurance athlete and you need specific nutrition strategies that will help you avoid the infamous "did not finish" (DNF), cross the finish line, or break through for a personal record.

I wrote this book not only as a Sports Dietitian but also as a competitive endurance athlete. I have competed in all types of endurance events since 1993 at all different distances and levels. I wrote this book thinking about the information I would want to know to achieve my goals. I hope you enjoy reading it as much as I enjoyed writing it!

1

Periodization

Chances are pretty good that if you are reading this, you classify yourself as some type of endurance athlete. That means that you have probably at least heard of the term periodization. It's that thing that athletes and coaches talk about when they discuss training.

WHAT IS PERIODIZATION?

Periodization is nothing more than separating your training year into different cycles and setting different goals for each cycle-goals that will get you to your key races in top shape (see Figure 1.1).

Periodization is a strategy that promotes an improvement in performance by varying training specificity, intensity, and volume throughout the year. By manipulating each of these variables with just the right blend of science and art, you can almost guarantee that you will race well. This chapter is not about how to set up your training program, as there are many books available that will help you do that. Instead, this chapter will provide you with basic information about periodization so you have some concrete knowledge about the concept and you can understand how your nutrition plan should complement each periodization cycle.

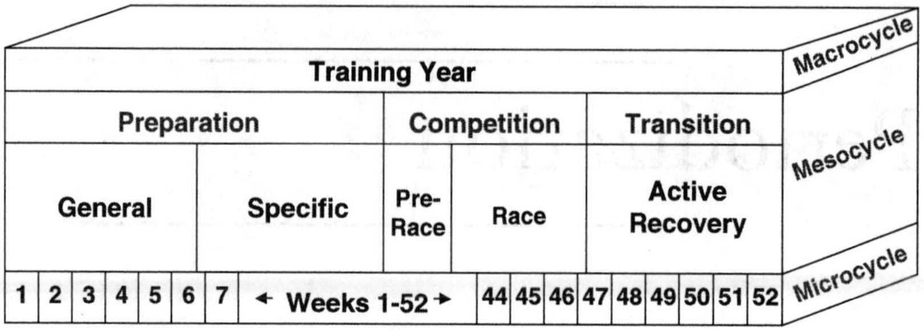

Training Year						
Preparation			Competition		Transition	Macrocycle
General		Specific	Pre-Race	Race	Active Recovery	Mesocycle
1 2 3 4 5 6 7	← Weeks 1-52 →		44 45 46 47 48 49 50 51 52			Microcycle

Figure 1.1 The Periodization Model

The History of Periodization

The periodization concept was discovered in the 1940s when Soviet sports scientists discovered that athletic performance was improved by varying the training stresses throughout the year rather than maintaining the same training from month to month. This led to the formal division of an athlete's year into cycles with differing training stresses. The East Germans and Romanians further developed this concept by applying goals to the various cycles, and the periodization concept was born.

The Components of Periodization

The traditional periodization concept breaks up your training program into specific cycles (see Figure 1.1). The largest cycle is a macrocycle, which is typically made up of one entire training year but may be longer for some athletes (e.g., those preparing for the Olympics). Within the macrocycle are smaller mesocycles, which can last several weeks or several months. The length of the mesocycles depends on what your goals are for the upcoming season, your strengths and weaknesses, and the number of races that you will be entering. Each mesocycle can then be divided into smaller microcycles that are typically one week in length but could last up to four weeks. Microcycles usually focus on your daily training session goals.

Whether you race to be competitive with yourself or are out for an age-group win or podium spot, you will still have the end goal of improving your fitness. There are many ways of getting there, but time and research tells us that adopting some type of periodization plan rather than random training-simply doing what you feel like doing each day-is the best way to achieve your goals. The terminology that most athletes and coaches use when talking about the major periodization cycles, or more specifically the mesocycles, are:

- Preparation
- Competition
- Transition

The Preparation Mesocycle

I say that these are the most agreed-upon terms across the board with athletes and coaches, but there are many variations on these mesocycles. For example, the preparation cycle is commonly referred to as "base training" and is sometimes broken down into "general" and "specific" cycles, corresponding to different training goals. During the general and specific periods of the preparation, or base training, mesocycle, your training intensity begins lower and gradually increases, while your training volume is moderate and slowly increases as the cycle progresses.

As a general rule, your preparation cycle should last 12–16 weeks with the goals of improving aerobic endurance, muscular strength, and flexibility. Long, slow distance (LSD) training is popular during this cycle, as is muscular endurance strength training. The weight training should include lifting lighter weights for higher repetitions in order to improve joint flexibility and tendon strength. Yoga or Pilates is also a good idea during this cycle to improve overall muscular flexibility.

The Competition Mesocycle

The competition mesocycle is sometimes referred to as the "intensity" or "build" cycle. It is sometimes broken down into "pre-race" and "race" cycles, each having a specific strength and/or speed focus. During the pre-race cycle, intensity is increasing and volume may be slowly decreasing, so that training intensity and volume intersect and cross This is where your sport-specific speed and strength are developed and improved.

In general, your pre-race cycle should last 8–12 weeks with the goals of improving your lactate threshold and VO_2 max. Hill repeats for cycling and running, lactate-threshold-specific intervals, VO_2-max-specific intervals, and strength training with an emphasis on explosive power (important for a handful of endurance athletes who rely more on anaerobic energy pathways needed in very short races and for sprint finishes) are the preferred training methods. Strength training is still important but since you already have a foundation of muscular endurance, you can spend the first part of this cycle developing muscular strength with heavier weights (e.g., "heavy" for endurance athletes, not what bodybuilders and powerlifters consider heavy) and fewer repetitions. You can then move toward more sport-specific exercises that include plyometrics such as bounds, squat jumps, medicine ball exercises, and arm swings during the second part of this cycle.

During the race phase of this mesocycle, your training intensity is still increasing while your training volume is decreasing to allow your body to recover in order to properly peak and taper for your races. A typical race season will last 12–24 weeks depending on where you live and where you travel to race. As a side note, it is important not to schedule your most important races, or "A" races, within 5–6 weeks of each other. You can have less important races sprinkled throughout your race season but try to focus on only a handful of "A" races to ensure proper physical recovery and to prevent injuries and overtraining.

The Transition Mesocycle

The transition cycle is sometimes referred to as "the off-season." This is a misnomer since the transition cycle is really an active recovery period, and you will still have sport-specific goals even though you are not competing. The main emphasis of the transition cycle initially should be having very little structure for your aerobic workouts. This provides your body and mind with a break from the structured training that you follow the other 50 or so weeks of the year. After the initial break of less-structured workouts, the transition cycle should be used to improve your weaknesses, so it really isn't as uneventful-or unimportant-as the term off-season implies.

As a general rule, the less-structured part of the transition cycle should last 2–4 weeks. It is important not to spend too long in the first part of this cycle since you don't want your overall physical fitness to decrease. After the first 2–4 weeks, the transition cycle generally lasts 4–12 weeks before the preparation cycle commences and the entire process begins over again.

As I mentioned previously, the focus for the transition cycle is improving your weaknesses. You should also spend more time doing less volume and more sport-specific drills. In swimming, these are the typical drills you do year-round but in the transition cycle they will make up about 50–75% of your swim workouts. In cycling, these are the one-legged pedaling drills, the high cadence drills, and the low heel pedaling drills. In running, these are the body position or hip flexion drills, high knees, butt kicks, and arm swings. Your workouts should be lower in total volume but higher in the amount of technique work. Remember, the goal of doing drill work is to teach your body how to perform movements the correct way.

There are many principles associated with periodization, but don't get too bogged down by the science. If you have a basic understanding of what periodization is, you can tailor it to your specific body and training program. The most important thing to remember is that each cycle should be set up to have specific physiological, psychological, and nutritional goals that will help you improve as an athlete. As long as you progress in a steady, logical way, making sure that your body is prepared for the next cycle, then you should be more than ready to race to your potential each year.

OVERTRAINING AND INJURY

I feel that I need to include this topic in this first chapter since most endurance athletes are infamous for training too much and not listening to their bodies. Another beneficial reason for following a training program that is periodized is for injury prevention. When athletes follow a random training program, there is more chance that the athlete will overdo one or more workouts and the risk for overtraining and injury become very high. This could result in an unplanned break or quite possibly in forfeiting the race season entirely. Recovery becomes extremely important during training, whether it is recovery days, weeks, or cycles. There is a limit to your capacity to endure and adapt to intense training. Once this threshold is crossed, your body fails to adapt and your performance declines rapidly. In fact, 10–20% of athletes who train intensively may fall prey to overtraining at some point during their endurance sport career.

The term *overtraining* itself is fraught with controversy and confusion. As established by the United States Olympic Committee and the American College of Sports Medicine's human performance summit, the following definitions are commonly used when talking about overtraining:

Overload: A planned, systematic and progressive increase in training with the goal of improving performance.

Overreaching: An unplanned, excessive overload in training with inadequate rest. Poor performance is observed in training and competition.

Overtraining: Untreated overreaching that results in chronic decreases in performance and impaired ability to train. This may require medical attention.

There are many causes associated with overtraining but the primary cause is a poorly planned training program. The biggest culprit is a rapid increase in your training volume and intensity combined with inadequate recovery and rest. Other types of stressors such as racing, environmental factors, psychosocial factors, and travel can increase the stress of training and contribute to overtraining, as can medical conditions and problems with nutrition.

If you find yourself fitting one of the categories of overreaching or overtraining, the smartest thing to do is rest. It may take weeks or even months, but unstructured activity is the best remedy to help you recover and get back in condition to train. In most cases, if overreaching is caught early, you won't have to completely stop training, but you should reduce your training volume and intensity.

Signs of Overtraining

The physical signs include:

- Decreased performance
- Loss of coordination
- Prolonged recovery
- Elevated morning heart rate
- Headaches
- Loss of appetite
- Muscle soreness/tenderness
- Gastrointestinal disturbances
- Decreased ability to ward off infection (repeated bouts of illness)

Athletes can also experience non-physical symptoms such as:

- Depression
- Apathy
- Difficulty concentrating
- Emotional sensitivity
- Decreased self-esteem

Recovery

I touched on recovery a little when discussing overtraining but I'm addressing it again because recovery is crucial to your success as an endurance athlete. Not many endurance athletes know this but during your cycles of increased volume and intensity, your fitness level does not improve. In fact, it may actually decrease slightly due to the repeated physical stress that is placed on your body. It is only during planned recovery that includes less volume and intensity that your body actually improves its fitness; the body needs a chance to repair itself (see Figure 1.2).

Figure 1.2 shows a one-month mesocycle where training volume is steadily increased each week. You can see that as volume

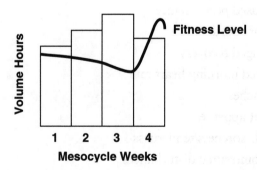

Figure 1.2 Progressive Build and Recovery Weeks of a Mesocycle

increases, fitness level slowly starts to decrease. However as soon as the recovery week begins, your body rejuvenates itself and recovers from the previous three weeks of training. The result is an increase in fitness.

By following a model similar to this one, a 3:1 build-to-recover model, you can reap the rewards of improved performance without injury or overtraining. There is nothing sacred about using the 3:1 build-to-recover model. Choose the right number of build cycles to fit your training plan and lifestyle but be sure to include recovery weeks often. If you are using a 3:1 build-to-recover model and you find that you are not able to complete your workouts in the third build week or that you are overly fatigued, you may have to choose a 2:1 model to accommodate your physical needs. Remember, when you are deciding which model to use, be sure to account for other stressors or time commitments that will increase your stress such as career, family, or social engagements.

As well as providing you with the energy you need to train, proper nutrition can help you avoid overtraining injuries and speed recovery. The chapters that follow will address how your nutrition plan can complement your periodization program. Training appropriately and eating appropriately will help you become a better and healthier athlete no matter what your event.

2

Nutrients for Life

As you read in the introduction, this book is not another sports nutrition book like the others that are on the market. This book is intended to complement those books and provide you with the unique information that you need to be successful in your endurance sport competition. To do this, you need to know the right nutrients to eat and drink in the right amounts at the right times of your training cycle.

This chapter will be an overview of the six essential nutrients. It will provide you with the base knowledge level needed to understand the concepts provided in the following chapters, which focus on the specifics of nutrition periodization. These concepts are cutting-edge and you may or may not have heard of them in the context that you will see them in this book. Read this material carefully and make sure you understand each key concept fully before moving on to the next. The process will be well worth it. If you apply the concept of nutrition periodization into your yearly training program, you will attain a new level of performance—I can almost guarantee it!

THE SIX ESSENTIAL NUTRIENTS

The basics of nutrition science will be the focus of Chapter 2. There are six essential nutrients that we need to have in order to maintain life and support training. They are:

1. Carbohydrates
2. Protein
3. Fat
4. Water
5. Vitamins
6. Minerals

Keep in mind that if you understand the basics of energy contribution from and digestion of carbohydrates, protein, and fat, then you will have a much better understanding of how certain foods will affect your body during training and racing. In this chapter, you will learn a few key scientific principles that will help you to properly fuel your body during training for competition. We will cover each of the essential nutrients listed above in some detail in the material that follows. Although not one of the essential nutrients, fiber—a form of undigestable carbohydrate that is an important part of a well-balanced diet that can affect performance—will also be discussed.

Before we get started with the nutrients, I will provide an overview of the digestive system since disturbances here are the main cause of problems during training and racing. How many times have you had stomach sloshing or repeated bouts of diarrhea during a long run? It could be the type of drink, bar, or gel you used or when you used it; either way I can almost guarantee at some point in your endurance sport career, you have experienced gastrointestinal (GI) distress, and you may experience it again. Having a base knowledge level of how foods pass through your system may help you better prepare your digestive system for competition and prevent GI distress in the future.

DIGESTION BASICS

After you eat or drink something, your brain and body release hormones that direct the digestive system to digest and absorb the foodstuff. The digestive system itself is a flexible, muscular tube extending from the mouth through the throat, esophagus, stomach, small intestine, large intestine, and rectum to the anus. It has a total length of about 26 feet.

The digestive tract is composed of the following organs and each has a role in food digestion:

- Mouth—chews and mixes food with saliva
- Esophagus—passes food to the stomach
- Stomach—adds acid, enzymes, and fluid and churns, mixes, and grinds food to a liquid mass
- Small intestine—secretes enzymes that digest carbohydrates, fat, and protein and absorbs nutrients into the blood
- Large intestine or colon—reabsorbs water and minerals and passes waste and some water to the rectum
- Rectum—stores waste prior to elimination
- Anus—holds rectum closed and opens to allow elimination

The digestive tract also has accessory organs that aid in digestion:

- Salivary glands—donate a starch-digesting enzyme and a trace of fat-digesting enzyme
- Liver—manufactures bile that helps break down fat
- Gallbladder—stores bile until it is needed
- Bile duct—carries the bile to the small intestine
- Pancreatic duct—carries pancreatic juice to the small intestine
- Pancreas—manufactures enzymes to digest all energy-yielding nutrients and releases bicarbonate, which neutralizes stomach acid that enters the small intestine

CARBOHYDRATES

Carbohydrates are the ultimate source of energy for our bodies and our brain. In fact, our brain relies on about 95% carbohydrates to function properly. In addition to providing energy, carbohydrates also play a protein-sparing role. When glycogen (the storage form of carbohydrates) levels become low, the body begins to make glucose from protein and fat. This is not a good thing because we want to maintain our muscle protein stores. In addition, the process of turning fat into carbohydrates is very inefficient (this process actually uses energy to make energy) and slow.

This book will not specify the amount of carbohydrates (or protein or fat) that you should eat on a daily basis, because this depends highly upon the specific training cycle that you are in. This topic will be discussed in detail in the Nutrition Periodization chapter. In that chapter you will learn how to calculate specifically how much you will need for each of your periodization cycles and how to customize these numbers based on your performance, health, and body weight goals. This chapter will provide the fundamentals of nutrition needed to apply nutrition periodization to your training cycle.

Each gram of carbohydrate provides four calories. The average athlete can only store approximately 1,600–1,800 calories from carbohydrates in their muscles, liver, and blood. This is one of the main reasons why athletes need to consume carbohydrates at such frequent intervals during training and racing.

Carbohydrate digestion begins in the mouth. Carbohydrates then pass through the stomach on their way to the small intestine. It is in the small intestine where all carbohydrates (except fiber) enter the bloodstream and are sent to the liver for further breakdown and delivery to the cells or to be stored as glycogen.

Types of Carbohydrates

There are two main classifications of carbohydrates: simple and complex, each with different chemical structures.

Simple carbohydrates, often called simple sugars, are made up of short chains of sugars; and are classified as mono-, di-, and oligosaccharides. Complex carbohydrates, or complex sugars, are made up of longer chains, also called polysaccharides, and include starch and fiber. In general terms, as a sugar (carbohydrate) becomes more complex it is more difficult to digest and its digestion takes longer.

Simple Carbohydrates

Monosaccharides include glucose, fructose, and galactose and are the simplest form of carbohydrate. They are made up of one simple sugar molecule and are the easiest to digest.

Disaccharides include sucrose, lactose, and maltose. These are made up of two monosaccharides and are not as easy to digest as monosaccharides.

Oligosaccharides by definition contain three to nine monosaccharides and include maltodextrins, corn syrup, and high-fructose corn syrup and are most often manufactured. Artificially sweetened foods often contain oligosaccharides. These take longer to digest than either of the above.

Complex Carbohydrates

Polysaccharides are often referred to as complex carbohydrates and include starch and fiber. They are made up of long, complex chains of sugars and require more complex mechanisms for digestion than simple carbohydrates.

Sources of Carbohydrates

Carbohydrates are found in the following foods:

- Breads
- Grains
- Starches
- Legumes

- Beans
- Fruits
- Vegetables
- Dairy products

Serving Sizes

Bread, Cereal, and Pasta (80 calories per serving)

- 1 slice of bread
- 2 slices of lite or reduced-calorie bread
- 1/2 English muffin or hamburger bun
- 3/4 cup cold cereal
- 1/3 cup rice, barley, couscous, or legumes
- 1/2 cup pasta, bulgur, sweet potato, corn, or green peas

Vegetables (25 calories per serving)

- 1 cup raw leafy vegetables
- 1/2 cup other vegetables, cooked or chopped raw
- 3/4 cup vegetable juice

Fruit (60 calories per serving)

- 1 small fruit (banana, apple, orange, or nectarine)
- 1 medium peach
- 1 kiwi
- 1/2 cup chopped, cooked, or canned fruit
- 1/2 cup unsweetened juice
- 1/2 grapefruit or mango
- 4 teaspoons jelly or jam

Carbohydrates and the Endurance Athlete

There is quite a debate regarding how much carbohydrate endurance athletes need to eat. To better understand this, it is important to first understand what our body needs based on the intensity of exercise that we do.

The predominant energy system utilized by endurance athletes is aerobic with brief, intermittent involvement of anaerobic energy systems. Your actual energy expenditure depends on the intensity, duration, and type of exercise. Exercise intensities may range between 50–90% VO_2 max for events lasting 4–24 hours, with total energy expenditures ranging from 5,000–10,000 calories per day in an event such as an Ironman. Multi-day events, such as adventure racing, could easily exceed 10,000 calories per day.

In a typical endurance event lasting longer than 4 hours, the exercise intensity averages ≤65% VO_2 max, and fat will be your primary fuel source. However, if you increase your exercise intensity, racing at an exercise intensity ≥75% VO_2 max, carbohydrate will be your primary fuel source.

The extreme daily energy expenditure of endurance events requires a significant contribution from all macronutrient energy sources. Although fat oxidation provides the greatest relative contribution to energy expenditure at low to moderate intensities, with a peak around 64% VO_2 max, and becomes increasingly important as an energy source as the length of exercise increases, exercise can only be maintained for prolonged periods without the onset of fatigue if sufficient carbohydrate is available. Despite the reports of successful performance following high-fat diets, sports dietitians continue to recommend that carbohydrate should be the main fuel consumed during endurance events to supplement muscle and liver glycogen stores and maintain blood glucose concentrations. While protein has made its way onto center stage as of late, it does not contribute significantly to energy levels in an endurance event unless carbohydrate stores and intakes are low. In this case, amino acid oxidation has been shown to contribute up to 15% of total energy, but the contribution of amino acid oxidation decreases to 5% when overall energy intake is adequate. Following the current guidelines of high carbohydrate consumption before and during an endurance event will minimize the contribution from protein as an energy source.

At rest, our bodies utilize carbohydrates for approximately 35% of its energy (60% from fat and 2–5% from protein). That is, it gets 35% of the energy it needs from carbohydrates and 60% from fat. As we begin to exercise lightly, say on our long slow training days, our bodies utilize about 40% carbohydrates (55% fat and 2–5% protein). Intervals, or high-intensity sprint-type exercise such as hill repeats, utilize about 95% carbohydrates (3% fat and 2% protein). The intensity that most of us race at, and train at if you are in an intensity or build cycle, utilizes about 70% carbohydrates (15% fat and 5–8% protein).

As you can see, carbohydrates are an important part of the training diet for endurance athletes and should be included in different amounts during different times of the year based on training. You will learn more about this in the Nutrition Periodization chapter but I want to make sure that you have a good understanding of why you need to supply your body with carbohydrates on a consistent basis.

PROTEIN

Contrary to popular belief, protein does not build muscle. Protein provides your muscles with the amino acids they need to *resynthesize* and *rebuild* new muscle cells. To illustrate this point, try sitting on the couch for a month consuming a protein supplement drink and eating a high-protein diet in hopes of building muscle (take this figuratively, please!). What you would find at the end of the month is that you had not built muscle because your muscles had not been overloaded with an external stimulus, such as weights, in any way. What would happen is that you would gain weight because the extra calories that you eat from protein would not be burned and would be stored as fat.

In your body, protein plays key roles in many areas, including:

- Enzymes—some proteins, known as enzymes, facilitate needed chemical reactions
- Hormones—some hormones, which regulate body processes, are proteins, are made from proteins, or require proteins in order to function
- Antibodies—proteins form the immune systems molecules that fight disease
- Fluid and electrolyte balance—proteins help to maintain the fluid and mineral composition of various body fluids
- Acid-base balance—proteins help maintain the acid-base balance (pH) of various body fluids by acting as buffers
- Energy—proteins provide some of the fuel for the body's energy needs
- Transportation—proteins help transport needed substances, such as fat, minerals and oxygen around the body
- Blood clotting-proteins provide the netting on which blood clots are built
- Structural components—proteins form integral parts of most body structures such as skin, tendons, ligaments, membranes, muscles, organs, and bones

Each gram of protein provides four calories. Unlike carbohydrate, after proteins are broken down into amino acids, many different things can happen to them. To understand the different fates that protein can meet in the body, it is important to first understand what makes up a protein. A protein is made up of amino acids. Each amino acid consists of an amine group (which is the nitrogen containing part), a carbon atom with a side-chain, and an acid. Each amino acid has a specific sidechain that gives it its identity and chemical nature. Amino acids can be used to build new proteins or other needed compounds (such as the vitamin niacin).

If the body has a surplus of amino acids and energy, the carbon backbone of the amino acid gets converted to fat and the nitrogen is excreted in the urine. This is why overdoing it on protein supplements is not beneficial—if you already have a good store of amino acids (which most athletes do), the remaining protein will be stored as fat.

Amino acids can be:

- Used to make other amino acids or other necessary compounds as mentioned above
- Converted to energy and used as fuel (during times of very long duration exercise and inadequate carbohydrate intake)
- Stored as fat (in times of eating too much protein)

The protein from food that you eat travels to the stomach where your stomach acid separates the protein strands into shorter strands and amino acids. These then travel to the small intestine where they are broken down further and absorbed into the blood for delivery to the cells in need of amino acids.

Types of Proteins

The two types of proteins are essential and non-essential. By definition, essential proteins provide all of the amino acids that our body cannot make—those that we need to obtain through food. These proteins are found in abundance in any animal product such as meat, fish, and dairy products, and in soy products and some grains such as quinoa. Nonessential proteins provide the amino acids that our body can make. These proteins are found in foods such as legumes, seeds and nuts, grains, and vegetables.

The essential amino acids are:

- Histidine
- Isoleucine
- Leucine
- Lysine
- Methionine
- Phenylalanine
- Threonine

- Tryptophan
- Valine

Nonessential amino acids are:

- Alanine
- Arginine
- Asparagine
- Aspartic acid
- Cysteine
- Glutamic acid
- Glutamine
- Glycine
- Proline
- Serine
- Tyrosine

Sources of Protein

Protein is found in the following foods:

- Meat products
- Dairy products
- Nuts
- Soy products
- Vegetables
- Grains

Serving Sizes

Fat Free and Very Low Fat Milk and Yogurt (90 calories per serving)

- 1 cup fat free or 1% milk
- 3/4 cup plain nonfat or low fat yogurt
- 1 cup artificially sweetened yogurt

Very Lean Protein (35 calories per serving)

- 1 ounce turkey or chicken breast (no skin)
- 1 ounce fish fillet (flounder, sole, cod, etc.), canned tuna in water, or shellfish (clams, lobster, shrimp, scallop)
- 3/4 cup cottage cheese, nonfat or low fat
- 2 egg whites
- 1/4 cup egg substitute
- 1/2 cup cooked beans (counts as one starch also)

Lean Protein (55 calories per serving)

- 1 ounce chicken or turkey (dark meat)
- 1 ounce salmon, swordfish, or herring
- 1 ounce lean beef (roast beef, London broil, or tenderloin), veal, lamb, or pork
- 1 ounce low fat cheese or lunch meat
- 2 medium sardines

Medium Fat Proteins (75 calories per serving)

- 1 ounce beef, corned beef, ground beef, pork chop
- 1 whole egg
- 1/4 cup ricotta cheese
- 4 ounces tofu (this is a very heart healthy choice)

FAT

The fats in foods and in our bodies fall into three classes. About 95% are triglycerides. The other two types are phospholipids (lecithin is one example) and sterols (cholesterol is the sterol most people know).

On average, our bodies have approximately 80,000 calories stored as fat. Sounds promising for the endurance athlete, doesn't it? Remember though, at higher intensity exercise, our bodies only utilize 3–15% energy from fat. The most energy we derive from fat is the 60% we utilize when we are at rest. The important lesson here is that it is not necessary to consume more fat in your diet to achieve better performance.

Fat is essential for body processes such as body insulation, internal organ protection, nerve transmission, and probably most importantly, metabolizing fat-soluble vitamins (A, D, E, and K). While a high-fat diet is detrimental to health, a diet too low in fat could potentially cause health problems also. The American Heart Association recommends that less than 30% of your total calories be from fat, but there is not a lower limit of fat intake since it depends on the specific person and any health-related issues.

One gram of fat has nine calories, which is more than two times the amount of calories per gram than carbohydrates or protein provide. Fat could potentially provide us with a large amount of energy if we were to always exercise at low intensity. But since we do not exercise at a low intensity all of the time, we must rely mainly on carbohydrates when exercise intensity increases.

We have the ability to store much more fat than carbohydrates because carbohydrates hold water and are quite bulky. Fat cells, on the other hand, pack tightly together and store much more energy in a smaller area. Fat has more "bang for your buck" in terms of energy but that isn't necessarily a good thing from a health or performance perspective. The non-healthy fats in our body cause serious health issues, such as heart disease and high cholesterol, and having more stored fat results in a higher body weight, which is detrimental to both health and performance. Eating the right amount and the right kinds of fat is the key to maximizing our health and performance.

The digestion of fat begins in the mouth just as it does for carbohydrates. Fat then travels to the stomach where it separates from other compounds and floats on top. Fat does not mix with the stomach fluids so very little digestion takes place in the stomach. From the stomach, it enters the small intestine where it mixes with bile and pancreatic juices, which break the fat down into smaller particles. These smaller particles are then absorbed into the bloodstream.

Types of Fats

There are two classifications of fats: saturated and unsaturated. Unsaturated fats have three additional subcategories: monounsaturated, polyunsaturated, and trans fats. Saturated fats are typically solid at room temperature, like butter, and unsaturated fats are typically liquid at room temperature, like olive oil. Chemically, saturated fats have most of their fatty acids saturated with hydrogen. Unsaturated fats have one or more fatty acids that are unsaturated. This difference in chemical structure makes a big difference when it comes to how these fats affect our health.

Saturated fats (SFA) often have the term *unhealthy* associated with them because they have a negative impact on heart health and could contribute to cardiovascular disease. Because these types of fats are not beneficial to our health, I recommend that no more than 10% of your total calories come from saturated fat.

The unsaturated fats, specifically mono- and poly-, are much better for health because they have positive effects on cardiovascular health.

Monounsaturated fats (MUFA) can be found in some oils (see Table 2.1), such as canola and olive, as well as from foods such as avocados, olives, and nuts. Polyunsaturated fats (PUFA) can be found in oils such as flaxseed and safflower, and from foods such as fish, walnuts, and flax products. Monounsaturated fats should make up about 10–15% of your total daily calories and polyunsaturated fats should make up about 10% of your total daily calories.

While trans fats are classified technically as an unsaturated fat, there is nothing healthy about them. Trans fats are polyunsaturated oils that are hardened by hydrogenation. Manufactured

Table 2.1
Fat Composition of Some Oils

Oil	SFA	MUFA	PUFA
Canola	minimal	~60%	~35%
Flaxseed	minimal	~20%	~75%
Safflower	~10%	~15%	~75%
Vegetable	~10%	~40%	~50%
Sunflower	~15%	~20%	~65%
Olive	~15%	~75%	~10%
Soybean	~15%	~25%	~60%
Corn	~20%	~30%	~50%
Peanut	~20%	~40%	~40%
Palm	~50%	~40%	~10%
Palm kernel	~90%	~10%	minimal
Coconut	~95%	~5%	minimal

hydrogenated oils, in addition to being saturated, often have altered chemical shapes as well. This change in shape results in a higher risk for heart disease because trans fats can cause an increase in low-density lipoprotein (LDL or the "bad" cholesterol) and a decrease in high-density lipoprotein (HDL or the "good" cholesterol). Because of the chemical changes to these fats they are worse for you than natural saturated fats like butter. Trans fats should be completely eliminated from the diet if possible. Most food labels do not have trans fats listed on them yet so you need to look at the ingredients list for "partially hydrogenated oils." If it says this on the label you know a product contains trans fats. Stay away from these products or limit the amount that you eat. Almost all processed foods and snacks have trans fat in them so beware and read the ingredients list.

Essential Fatty Acids

In the polyunsaturated fat category, there are two additional fats that are very popular in the press. Omega-6 and omega-3 fatty acids are essential polyunsaturated fatty acids (PUFA) or essential fatty acids (EFA), which cannot be made by the body's cells. The cells cannot convert one fat to another. Therefore these fats must be provided by the diet.

Essential fatty acids (EFA) have many very important health functions:

- Blood pressure regulation
- Blood clot formation
- Regulation of blood lipids
- Acting like hormones
- Assisting the immune response
- Decreasing the inflammation response to injury and infection

In addition, EFAs serve as structural parts of cell membranes, constitute a major part of the lipids of the brain and nerves, and are essential to normal growth and vision in infants and children.

The omega-6 fatty acid, linoleic acid, is found in many popular vegetable oils (see Table 2.2) and is consumed in excess in our society. This could lead to significant health problems because a high consumption of linoleic acid can lead to an increase in the production of eicosanoids that are involved in inflammatory, cardiovascular, and immunological diseases.

The omega-3 fatty acid, alpha-linolenic acid, is not as abundant as linoleic acid but is available in certain foods and oils (see Table 2.2). Unfortunately, because it is not as easy to locate as linoleic acid, alpha-linolenic acid is not consumed in large amounts in our society. This omega-3 fat may have very positive health outcomes including the following:

- Decreasing risk of coronary artery disease
- Decreasing hypertension
- Improving insulin sensitivity for individuals with Type 2 diabetes
- Reducing tenderness in joints for individuals with rheumatoid arthritis
- Assisting with proper development of the brain's cerebral cortex

Table 2.2
Approximate EFA Content of Some Popular Oils

Oil	g Omega-3 per 100 g Oil	Oil	g Omega-6 per 100 g Oil
Flax/Linseed oil	58	Safflower oil	74
Flax/Linseeds	15–30	Grapeseed oil	68
Walnut oil	11.5	Sunflower oil	63
Canola/ Rapeseed oil	7	Walnut oil	58
		Soybean oil	51
Soybean oil	7	Corn oil	50
Wheatgerm oil	5	Sesame oil	43
		Canola/ Rapeseed oil	20
		Flax/Linseed oil	0

- Assisting with proper retina formation for proper vision
- Decreasing inflammatory disorders
- Protecting against stroke caused by plaque buildup and blood clots
- Lowering triglycerides and raising HDL levels

Omega-6 and omega-3 essential fatty acids are best consumed in a ratio of 3:1 to maximize positive health benefits. Unfortunately, the ratio that exists in modern Western diets ranges from 10:1 up to 30:1.

Eating cold-water fish (mackerel, salmon, tuna) 3–4 times per week and increasing the consumption of flax products (flax meal and oil) is a good way to increase your consumption of omega-3 fats.

Sources of Fat

Fat is found in the following foods:

- Snack foods such as cookies and potato chips
- Butter
- Lard

- Animal products
- Dairy products
- Nuts
- Oils
- Mayonnaise
- Shortening
- Salad dressing

Serving Sizes

Fat (45 calories per serving)

- 1 teaspoon oil, butter, stick margarine, or mayonnaise
- 1 tablespoon reduced-fat margarine or mayonnaise, salad dressing, or cream cheese
- 2 tablespoons lite cream cheese
- 1/8 avocado
- 8 large black olives
- 10 large stuffed green olives
- 1 slice bacon

WATER

Of the six nutrients essential to life, water is by far the most important. Water makes up about 60–75% of total body weight. Drinking too little water or losing too much through sweating can inhibit your ability to exercise.

Not only does water keep our bodies hydrated, it also acts in the blood as a transport mechanism, eliminates metabolic waste products in urine, dissipates heat through sweat, helps to digest food, lubricates joints, and cushions organs. Water is an essential nutrient that is crucial to survival as well as athletic performance.

I know you have heard the saying, "Drink eight glasses of water per day". Well, it does not hold true any longer. Recent research has shown that the fluid needs of individuals differ greatly and the general recommendation to drink eight glasses of water per day is not applicable for some people. So how much water should you drink on a daily basis? Let me first explain a little about what drives you to drink, so you have an understanding about what is happening inside your body before I answer that question.

Thirst, defined as a conscious awareness of the desire for water and other fluids, usually controls water intake. The sensation of thirst is triggered by abnormally high, concentrated body fluids. When you sweat, you lose significant amounts of water from your body, including your blood. The remaining blood becomes more concentrated and has, for example, an abnormally high sodium level. This triggers the thirst mechanism and increases your desire to drink. To quench your thirst, you must replace the water losses and bring the blood back to its normal concentration.

Scientifically, this makes sense. However, you should not trust your thirst mechanism alone. If you only drink water when your body tells you that you are thirsty, then you are already dehydrated before you begin to drink, and you begin playing the catch-up game of re-hydration. This is because it takes much longer to re-hydrate yourself than it does to maintain your hydrated state. And since you are most likely training at least 4–6 days per week, if you go into a workout dehydrated, it will significantly impact your performance, no matter the duration or intensity.

Yet another problem that you have as an athlete is that thirst can be blunted by exercise or overridden by the mind. Your body will usually only "tell" you to replace two-thirds of your sweat losses. Being one-third behind in fluid consumption is significant, especially if you are trying to do two-a-day workouts. How can you expect your body to function properly if your hydration tank is only two-thirds full? So we return to the question, how much water do you need to drink each day and how do you do it?

Recent research has proven that the best way to monitor your own hydration status is by the color of your urine. What this means is that throughout the day, with the exception of your morning pit stop, your urine should be no darker than the color of straw (pale yellow) or even clear. Following this rule will ensure that you are hydrated throughout the day. From my experience, allowing your urine color to dictate how much water you drink is highly accurate, and a better method of hydration control than thirst since you cannot rely on your thirst mechanism throughout the day to maintain hydration. Make a concerted effort to take in as many fluids as necessary to ensure that your urine is a clear to pale yellow color.

You can do this very easily by taking a water bottle or closed container of water with you wherever you go, even into meetings. I have noticed that athletes are less likely to drink often if they choose an open cup or glass because it is not portable. You should already have an abundance of water bottles. Make sure you keep one at work, one in the car, and have a few of them always ready in the refrigerator so that they are easy to grab anytime.

Fear not if you are an athlete who just doesn't like drinking water. Another great way to meet your daily fluid needs is by eating the right foods! Certain foods, such as fruits and vegetables, have a large amount of water in them. Your fluid needs do not need to be met from water alone. You can also stay hydrated with other beverages such as iced tea or lemonade and it has been found that the caffeine in some of these drinks is not as dehydrating as once thought.

VITAMINS

Vitamin supplements are big news these days. Everywhere you look there is a new company coming out with a "new" vitamin supplement that they claim is different from their competitors'.

This is simply not true. There are a few things that you should be aware of before choosing a vitamin supplement and I will discuss those in Chapter 6. In this chapter I will provide a clear explanation of what vitamins are, what they do in our bodies, and how to get them from foods.

Vitamins are metabolic catalysts that regulate biochemical reactions within the body. To date, 13 vitamins have been discovered, each with a specific function. What is important to note is that there is no scientific research that proves that extra vitamins offer a competitive edge. Obviously, if you have a vitamin deficiency, a vitamin supplement can help to correct that; however, vitamin deficiencies are usually related to a larger medical problem that needs attention. Keeping this in mind, some vitamins are stored in the body in large amounts (vitamins A, D, E, and K) and others in smaller amounts (vitamins B and C), so it is virtually impossible for a nutritional deficiency to happen overnight.

So, does endurance exercise increase the body's vitamin needs? For most situations the answer is no because, remember, vitamins are only catalysts that are needed for metabolic processes to occur. Vitamins do not provide energy. There is no evidence that vitamins improve performance in athletes who are adequately nourished. Another important point is that endurance athletes tend to eat more because of their increased activity. Thus, endurance athletes consume more vitamins from food since they are eating more.

There are a few people who are at a higher risk for nutritional deficiencies and may consider taking a daily multivitamin. These include:

- Athletes who are eating less than 1200–1500 calories per day
- Athletes who are allergic to certain foods
- Athletes who are lactose intolerant, because this could result in low amounts of riboflavin and calcium
- Athletes who are pregnant

- Athletes who are contemplating pregnancy; folic acid, iron, and calcium are important during conception and pregnancy
- Athletes who are complete vegetarians; vegetarianism could result in low amounts of vitamins B_{12} and D, riboflavin, iron, and zinc

The bottom line is that as an endurance athlete, it is a good idea to try to get your vitamins from foods first. However since a "perfect" diet does not exist, taking a daily multivitamin that does not exceed 100% of the recommended daily allowance (RDA) of the vitamins may be beneficial. Remember though, each person is different and you should consult a registered dietitian specializing in sports nutrition and endurance athletes to determine if you have nutritional deficiencies. Here is an overview of the different vitamins, their functions, and food sources (the foods listed are not the only ones where the vitamin is present, just the more common ones):

Vitamin A or Retinol (fat soluble)

- Necessary for healthy eyes and skin and the linings of the digestive and urinary tracts and the nose.
- Food sources include milk, dried apricots, squash, carrots, spinach, and fortified products.

Vitamin B_1 or Thiamin (water soluble)

- Helps transform carbohydrates into energy.
- Food sources include potatoes, fish, bananas, ham, chicken, bread, cereal, and enriched rice.

Vitamin B_2 or Riboflavin (water soluble)

- Necessary for energy release and for healthy skin, mucous membranes, and nervous system.
- Food sources include spinach, steak, cottage cheese, milk, oranges, apples, enriched bread, and enriched cereal.

Vitamin B₃ or Niacin (water soluble)

- Helps transform food into energy (metabolism); necessary for growth and for production of hormones.
- Food sources include tuna, potatoes, halibut, peas, cereal, corn, mushrooms, peanut butter, ground beef, and enriched bread.

Vitamin B₆ (water soluble)

- Necessary for synthesis and breakdown of amino acids; aids in metabolism of carbohydrates.
- Food sources include peanut butter, chick peas, chicken, spinach, cereal, potatoes, bananas, and lima beans.

Folic Acid (water soluble)

- Necessary for production of blood cells and a healthy nervous system.
- Food sources include spinach, broccoli, green beans, peas, lentils, asparagus, mushrooms, lima beans, and oranges.

Biotin (water soluble)

- Necessary for metabolism of carbohydrates, protein, and fat.
- Food sources include nuts, split peas, eggs, cauliflower, and mushrooms.

Pantothenic Acid (water soluble)

- Needed for metabolism of carbohydrates, protein, and fat.
- Food sources include eggs, peanuts, mixed vegetables, steak, fish, wheat germ, and broccoli.

Vitamin B₁₂ (water soluble)

- Needed for synthesis of red and white blood cells and for the metabolism of food.
- Food sources include chicken, meat, eggs, milk, and yogurt.

Vitamin C *(water soluble)*

- Necessary for healthy connective tissue, bones, teeth, and cartilage; enhances immune system.
- Food sources include bell peppers, broccoli, strawberries, oranges, potatoes, tomatoes, and kiwi.

Vitamin D *(fat soluble)*

- Needed for calcium and phosphorus metabolism and for healthy bones and teeth.
- Sources include milk, fortified milk, fortified cereal, and sunlight.

Vitamin E *(fat soluble)*

- Necessary for nourishing and strengthening cells; is an antioxidant.
- Food sources include sunflower oil, wheat germ, sunflower seeds, almonds, and whole-wheat grains.

Vitamin K *(fat soluble)*

- Necessary for blood clotting.
- Food sources include cabbage, spinach, broccoli, and kale.

MINERALS

Minerals are elements that combine in various ways to form structures of the body and regulate body processes. We get minerals from the foods we eat, but they are not a source of energy. The minerals magnesium, sodium, calcium, potassium, zinc, and iron are the more talked about minerals among endurance athletes because of their impacts on hydration and cramping, oxygen delivery, and immune system health. Here I will provide you an overview of each of these and other minerals, their functions, and food sources so you have a basic understanding of the importance of each.

Calcium

- Necessary for bone formation, enzyme reactions, and muscle contractions.
- Food sources include dairy products, green leafy vegetables, and beans.

Iron

- Necessary for hemoglobin formation, muscle growth and function, and energy production.
- Food sources include lean meat, beans, dried fruit, and some green leafy vegetables.

Magnesium

- Necessary for energy production, muscle relaxation, and nerve signal conduction.
- Food sources include grains, nuts, meats, and beans.

Sodium

- Necessary for nerve impulses, muscle action, and body fluid balance.
- Food sources include table salt. Sodium is also found in small amounts in most foods except for fruit.

Potassium

- Necessary for fluid balance, muscle action, and glycogen and protein synthesis.
- Food sources include bananas, orange juice, fruits, and vegetables.

Zinc

- Necessary for tissue growth and healing, immunity, and gonadal development.
- Food sources include meat, shellfish, oysters, and grains.

Copper

- Necessary for hemoglobin formation, energy production, and immunity.
- Food sources include whole grains, beans, nuts, dried fruit, and shellfish.

Selenium

- Necessary as an antioxidant, which protects against free radicals.
- Food sources include meat, seafood, and grains.

Chromium

- Necessary for glucose uptake as part of the glucose tolerance factor.
- Food sources include whole grains, meat, and cheese.

Manganese

- Necessary for bone and tissue development and fat synthesis.
- Food sources include nuts, grains, beans, tea, fruits, and vegetables.

Iodine

- Necessary for regulating metabolism.
- Food sources include iodized salt and seafood.

Fluoride

- Necessary for the formation of bones and tooth enamel.
- Food sources include fluoridated tap water, tea, coffee, rice, spinach, and lettuce.

Phosphorus

- Necessary for building bones and teeth; aids in metabolism.
- Food sources include meat, fish, dairy products, and carbonated drinks.

FIBER

The fibers of a plant form the supporting structures of the leaves, stems, and seeds. Most fiber passes through the digestive tract without providing any energy because our digestive enzymes cannot break them apart. In the digestive tract, fiber can do the following:

- Slow the absorption of nutrients
- Delay cholesterol absorption
- Bind bile for excretion
- Increase stool weight
- Stimulate bacterial fermentation, causing gas

The health benefits of eating a diet rich in fiber are great. Fiber:

- Possibly reduces the risk of heart disease and stroke because soluble fiber delays absorption of cholesterol and binds with bile to get the bad cholesterol out of the body
- Improves the body's handling of glucose and insulin so the risk of developing diabetes is lower
- Helps in maintaining body weight because a diet high in fiber can result in a feeling of fullness and thus can reduce the amount of food eaten
- Improves the health of the digestive tract by stimulating the muscles of the digestive tract so that they retain their tone thereby preventing the condition diverticulosis
- Helps to prevent constipation and hemorrhoids because insoluble fiber softens stools and regulates bowel movements

Why am I discussing fiber in a book for endurance athletes? Fiber is very healthy to have in abundance in your normal eating program, but at certain times of the year—before your major competition events—it may be feasible to follow a lower-fiber diet to improve your performance. Knowing what fiber is and what it does in your body will help you prevent major catastrophes during your races. I'll cover this in much more detail in Chapter 4.

Types of Fiber

Fiber can be soluble or insoluble. Soluble fiber includes gums, mucilages, pectins, psyllium, and some hemicelluloses. Insoluble fiber includes cellulose, lignin, and some hemicelluloses. Here is a breakdown of health benefits and food sources of each type.

Soluble

Health Benefits

- Lowers cholesterol
- Slows glucose absorption
- Slows transit of food
- Softens stools
- Is partly fermentable into fragments the body can use

Food Sources

- Barley
- Fruits
- Legumes
- Oats
- Oat bran
- Rye
- Seeds
- Vegetables

Insoluble

Health Benefits

- Softens stools
- Regulates bowel movements
- Speeds transit of materials through the small intestine
- Increases fecal weight and speeds its passage
- Reduces risk of diverticulosis, hemorrhoids, and appendicitis

Food Sources

- Brown rice
- Fruits
- Legumes
- Seeds
- Vegetables
- Wheat bran
- Whole grains

It is generally recommended that you eat 20–35 grams of fiber each day. Table 2.3 will help you determine how to effectively get enough fiber in your diet through the foods you eat.

SUMMARY

If you didn't notice, in this chapter I did not provide specific amounts of carbohydrates, protein, and fat for you to eat. Because nutritional needs differ depending on the athlete, I don't like to provide general guidelines such as percentages of total calories or ranges. Following general guidelines will not provide you with the specific amounts of nutrients that your body needs. Instead of providing general guidelines, this book will help you to be as accurate as possible in meeting your nutritional needs by configuring your diet based on your

Table 2.3
High-Fiber Favorites

Food	Portion Size	Fiber (g)
Banana	1 medium	2.4
Apple	1 medium	3.6
Orange	1 medium	2.9
Peach	1 medium	1.9
Prunes	6 medium	8.0
Carrots	1/2 cup	2.3
Corn	1/2 cup	3.6
Green peas	1/2 cup	3.6
Potato with skin	1 medium	2.5
Beans, cooked		
Lima	1/2 cup	4.5
Navy	1/2 cup	6.0
Kidney, Pinto	1/2 cup	6.7
Bran flakes	3/4 cup	4.0
Shredded wheat	1 biscuit	3.0
Air-popped popcorn	1 cup	1.0
Whole-wheat bread	1 slice	2.1
White bread	1 slice	0.4
Broccoli	1/2 cup	3.8
Spinach	1/2 cup	2.1
Zucchini	1/2 cup	1.6
Brown rice, cooked	1/2 cup	5.3
Oatmeal, dry	1/3 cup	2.8
Corn flakes	1 ounce	0.3

current body weight, body weight goals, and performance goals. This way you can develop a plan based on the amount of carbohydrate, protein, and fat that you need at specific times during your training. In Chapter 4, I will provide specific grams-per-unit-of-body-weight recommendations that are based on your specific training cycles, not on national population averages.

Practice sensible moderation and balance in the choices that you make so you do not overeat one nutrient compared to another. Practicing moderation, eating a wide variety of foods, and having a good amount of color in your daily eating program will ensure that you are eating all of the nutrients you need to maintain health and your endurance training and racing regimen.

3

Nutrition Periodization

Now that you realize the importance of having a structured training program that focuses on varying the volume and intensity of your training along with including recovery weeks, and you have learned the basic role of the nutrients and the importance of diet, it's time to go to the next step. In order to properly prepare yourself for endurance sport you must use physiological, psychological, and nutritional concepts (see Figure 3.1). Your physiological training will be structured based on your yearly periodization program and your psychological training will be developed through specific mental training work. In order to make the most out of your physiological and psychological training, you need to have a sound nutritional plan as well. The concept of nutrition in an overall training program will be the main focus of this chapter.

THE IMPORTANT ROLE OF NUTRITION

I know you believe that good nutrition is important, but I also know that you probably don't plan it with as much thought or detail as you do your physical training. Nutrition is the most commonly overlooked component in an endurance athlete's training program. At best most athletes concern themselves with

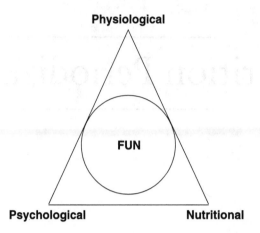

Figure 3.1 Three Cornerstones of Endurance Training

nutrition one week to a few days before their race or only during training sessions. This is fine if you just want to finish your race but it will not help you achieve peak performance and set new personal records.

Maintaining proper nutrition throughout the year will not make you stronger or faster in itself. However it will provide you with the correct amount and timing of nutrients so that you can improve your health, prevent illnesses, and change your body weight and composition—all with the end goal of improving your performance. Let's face it, one of the reasons we are endurance athletes is because exercise either helps regulate our body weight (meaning we don't have to worry about how much we eat because we will burn off the extra calories in our training) or it helps us achieve a desired body weight. And of course, to a certain extent, racing at a lower body weight without sacrificing power output, strength, or health will make you race faster. So treat nutrition with all the care you give your physical training. That is, plan, plan, and plan. As you will learn in this chapter, there are certain times of the year during your physical periodization cycles when your nutrition must change to supply the right mix of nutrients. There are other times when your nutrition needs to be the most important factor if you want to change your body weight for health or performance reasons.

Don't let nutrition take a back seat to your training. Your eating program supports your body so you are able to train, not the other way around. It is the missing link that you need to feel better after races and to beat your competition or set new personal records. Don't underestimate the power of periodizing your nutrition to support your training. If you neglect your nutrition, I guarantee it will come back and bite you!

PERIODIZATION AND NUTRITION PLANNING

Each periodization cycle that you follow requires a different mix of volume and intensity. With those changes to volume and intensity, come corresponding increases or decreases of stress on your body. In addition, there is a corresponding increase or decrease in the quantity and timing of carbohydrate, protein, fat, and fluids your body needs. I know that planning your training program can be quite a complex puzzle at times and it can be challenging to determine what the right mix of volume and intensity is for your body. The nutrition periodization concept is not meant to further complicate the matter. It is meant to provide your body with the needed energy and fluids at the right time to allow you to experiment with your physical training. In this way you can come to a conclusion regarding what works best for you body. If you don't have enough energy or you are dehydrated when you are trying different run intervals on the track or trying to figure out what speed or power output you should be riding on the bike to improve your lactate threshold, then you will not be able to determine your optimum training program and, therefore, you will never be as successful as you want to be.

While your nutrition periodization program does not need to be too complicated, you will have slightly different eating programs during each of your periodization cycles in order to match the energy (calories) you burn through training, create a negative energy balance for weight loss, or create a positive energy balance that focuses on carbohydrates to increase glycogen storage prior to a race.

Remember, each athlete is different so you should use the following recommendations as a starting point to begin planning your individual eating program and customize them based on your specific needs. Sports nutrition for endurance athletes is both a science and an art. I present the quantitative numbers that science has given us and use art to apply it to the different training cycles and specific goals and objectives. As you know, there is no one right eating program for everyone.

Nutrition Periodization Specifics

It has been recommended that during training or competition an endurance athlete's eating plan could include 5–19 grams of carbohydrate per kilogram of body weight, 1.2–3.0 grams of protein per kilogram of body weight, and 0.8–3.0 grams of fat per kilogram of body weight. The ranges are large because training and racing time and distance vary among endurance athletes. You could be racing a sprint triathlon, the Race Across America cycling race, or an adventure race. Each requires a different amount of time to finish and a different intensity to be sustained.

Keep in mind that it has been shown that the human body can absorb about 1 gram of carbohydrate per minute of moderately intense exercise, so the following are guidelines that you should first try in training and then customize to your body and your training and race needs. One gram of carbohydrate per minute is the equivalent of 60 grams per hour, which is 240 calories (the amount in about one energy bar or two energy gels) per hour.

As I mentioned before, nutrition periodization is not meant to be complicated or difficult. Nutrition periodization is meant to help you achieve peak health and performance by encouraging you to make slight changes in your nutrition during each of your physical periodization cycles. To help you make these changes, I use the same physical periodization cycles that were discussed in Chapter 1 and apply the specific nutrition periodization principles to each cycle so that it is easy for you to tie nutrition into your training cycle.

Figure 3.2 describes the concept of nutrition periodization in graphic form. You can see that there are specific macrocycle, mesocycle, and microcycle nutrition goals depending upon which training cycle you are in throughout the year.

Let's begin at the top with macrocycle nutritional goals and then get into the details of the meso- and microcycle nutritional goals.

MACROCYCLE NUTRITION GUIDELINES

There are some nutrition guidelines that I would like to include here that apply year-round no matter what type of endurance athlete you are or what training cycle you may be in at any given time. These guidelines are more about improving health than improving performance. However, better general health is correlated to an improvement in performance, so try to adopt these guidelines in

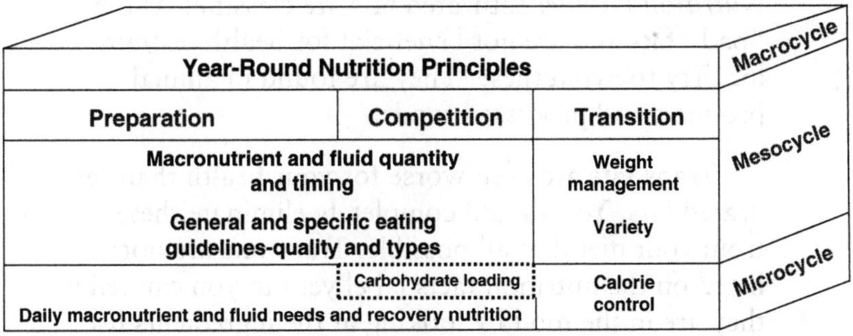

Figure 3.2. Nutrition Periodization

your daily eating program. Below, you will find specific needs and timing recommendations of nutrients with notes about each, what I term *nutrition nibbles*. These nibbles are meant to help you understand and apply each nutrition principle that is presented.

General and Specific Eating Guidelines for Good Health

- **Choose foods rich in beta-carotene, vitamin C, vitamin E, and zinc to support immune function.**

   Nutrition Nibble: Eating foods that have more phyto-chemicals (plant compounds that improve health and prevent disease) and nutrients will help keep your immune system strong. As an endurance athlete, you are constantly pushing the envelope with your volume and intensity of training, which can lead to getting sick quite often.

   Good sources of beta-carotene are carrots and sweet potatoes. Good sources of vitamin C are oranges, kiwis, strawberries, and grapefruit. Vitamin E can be found in nuts and green leafy vegetables. Zinc can be found in oysters, red meat, poultry, beans, nuts, whole grains, and dairy products.

- **Choose polyunsaturated and monounsaturated fats rather than saturated and trans fats.**

   Nutrition Nibble: Saturated fats are classified as the "bad" fats and are not beneficial for health or training. Try to avoid these. They are found in animal products and processed foods.

   Trans fats are even worse for your health than saturated fats. You should completely eliminate these from your diet if at all possible. Trans fats are not listed on the nutrition facts label yet but you can tell if they are in the food by looking at the ingredients list. If the label lists "partially hydrogenated" oil then you know the product has trans fat.

Mono- and polyunsaturated fats are the "good" fats and are beneficial for health. You can find monounsaturated fats in olives, avocados, and olive oil. Polyunsaturated fats can be found in salmon, mackerel, tofu, almonds, walnuts, flax products, and canola oil.

- **Think about taking a multivitamin that has no more than 100% Daily Value (DV) for nutrients.**

Nutrition Nibble: A multivitamin is okay to take but some vitamin brands contain ridiculously high levels of vitamins and minerals. The fat-soluble vitamins A, D, E, and K are stored in your body, so taking more of these may lead to developing toxic levels of them in the future. The water-soluble vitamins B and C aren't stored as much in the body but shouldn't be taken in excess either since excess cannot be "held in reserve". Keep an eye out for iron also. Overdoing iron intake can result in a pro-oxidation of cells inside your arteries (the exact opposite of what you want to happen). Thankfully, overloading on iron usually isn't a concern unless you are an athlete currently supplementing with iron.

Because you will get some of the vitamins and minerals from the food that you eat, try to keep the levels found in your multivitamin to a minimum. If you decide to take a multivitamin, I recommend one with no more than 100% Daily Value (DV) for the vitamins and minerals. Children's chewable vitamins are an inexpensive and effective choice and help you avoid going overboard on vitamins and minerals.

- **Keep a written 3–5 day food diary when eating habits are out of control.**

Nutrition Nibble: This is always a good habit to get into once a month or whenever you feel that you are going in the wrong direction with your nutrition.

Keeping a food diary forces you to pay attention not only to what foods you eat but, more importantly, how much you eat of them. It is a great way to keep you in balance and sometimes will help you avoid unnecessary or emotional/stress eating.

By keeping a food log when your nutrition and training are going well, you can also have a good reference in the future to look back on when you want to replicate the same positive responses, so keeping a food log should not only be done during times of "trouble".

- **Listen to cravings and satisfy them within reason.**

  Nutrition Nibble: If you crave a food, then by all means, eat it (barring any pre-existing health conditions that would result in the food having a negative effect), but always practice portion control and moderation. The trick is to only have a small amount of less-than-healthy foods. I know it is difficult, but a good strategy to overcome indulging too much is to either divide these craving foods into smaller portions such as baggies when you buy them or to have a plan of attack before reaching for the food. If you plan that you will only have two pieces, then you will be more likely to stick to that plan. If you don't have a plan, you will end up going back for seconds, thirds, and fourths. Cravings sometimes mean your body needs the nutrients in that food, so don't fight the urge, just be sensible and limit the quantity.

- **Don't restrict eating to a few food groups. Increase variety.**

  Nutrition Nibble: Endurance athletes are infamous for having high-carbohydrate diets and eating a lot of breads and grains. While there is certainly nothing wrong with this since carbohydrates are your main source of energy for training and racing, it is not the best habit to maintain from a nutrient-balance stand-point. If you overeat in one food group, the other food groups will suffer and you will not get all of the essential nutrients that your body needs. So mix it up and choose a variety of foods from all of the food groups. You can easily accomplish this by having lean proteins, color (fruits and vegetables), whole grains, and healthy fats at most meals.

- **Don't consume too much fat after a training session or a race.**

  Nutrition Nibble: Fat can slow the absorption of car-bohydrates and the nutritional recovery process. I know the cookies or pizza that are typically found in abundance at the finish line sound really good after a race, but you will speed your recovery and be able to train better the following day if you back off of the fat for the first 2–4 hours after exercise.

- **Don't take any nutritional supplement that is not com-pletely proven as efficacious and safe.**

  Nutrition Nibble: Taking a nutritional supplement without knowing its full effects could have an ergolytic (negative impact on performance) effect. It could also adversely affect your health. There are not many proven nutritional supplements that produce positive effects for endurance athletes. If you stick with sports drinks, energy gels, energy bars, recovery drinks, and multivitamins you should be able to meet all of your needs—and not get things you don't need.

  Please remember that some of the new drinks on the market touted as sports drinks contain certain herbs that are not the best to drink during exercise. Carbohydrates, fluid, and electrolytes (mainly sodium) are the main nutrients that our bodies need during exercise, not additional herbs or additives.

- **You are unique so don't eat the same as a friend or family member just because it works for them.**

  Nutrition Nibble: Nutrition is highly individualized depending on your health, medical and family history, current fitness level, body weight goals, and performance-related goals. Your nutrition plan should be as individualized as your training program is.

- **Don't overeat.**

  Nutrition Nibble: Endurance athletes usually do not have this problem because the calories that are being burned from training balance out the calories that are being eaten. However, if you are injured or are in an active recovery or transition mesocycle, you should decrease the amount of calories you eat. Your body has developed a routine and at certain times, you are programmed to eat. When you are not training hard or racing, try to avoid eating out of habit and eat only when you are physiologically hungry. You will know when you are truly hungry because you will begin to have stomach pangs.

  I have seen far too many athletes who fall into this category and simply forget or do not pay attention to their nutrition during times when they are training less. Don't fall prey to this mistake. Weight gain is easy; weight loss is much harder and when done at the wrong time of the year, can have a negative impact on your training.

- **Don't worry about consuming more protein.**

  Nutrition Nibble: Most athletes consume at least 15% of their total calories as protein on a daily basis. In fact, research studies have shown that when people are given access to a buffet-style meal, they typically average about 15% of their total calories from protein.

Only if you are participating in a vigorous strength training program focused on improving lean muscle mass and are in the gym at least four times per week, will you possibly need a little more protein to support the new muscle tissue that is being formed.

The one exception is the endurance athlete who is completely vegan and does not eat any animal products whatsoever. It has been my experience that the seasoned vegan athlete knows how to properly build their eating program with just the right amount of carbohydrates, protein (from vegetable sources), and fat so this would really only apply to the athlete who has just become vegan. If this is the case, consult a registered dietitian to get you started on the right foot.

MESOCYCLE AND MICROCYCLE NUTRITION GUIDELINES

Now that you have the overall nutrition goals for the year, let's look at the specific guidelines for each of your meso- and microcycles. This information will be used on a daily basis to help support your training, but will also need to be applied to your training weeks to months in advance. Remember, the "new school" sports nutrition plans are those that are planned weeks to months in advanced rather than only in the days leading up to a big training day or race.

The Preparation Mesocycle (aka the Base Cycle)   A.

This is where it all begins: the start of a new journey to race season. You are just coming off of your transition cycle and you are slowly building up your volume but keeping your intensity low to make sure you ease into more intense training again without injury. Your physiological goals are to improve your cardiorespiratory system in order to be ready for the intensity or speed cycles that will come in the following months. During this base cycle, you may also be trying to lose weight. That is fine to do in the beginning of a 12–16-week preparatory cycle, but don't try to actively lose weight too close to your intensity/build cycle as it may have a negative impact on your training. By actively losing weight I mean that you are making a concerted effort to take in fewer calories or burn more calories each day. You may experience weight loss throughout your intensity/build and race cycles but you will not be actively seeking it. It will happen because you will be burning many more calories than you are taking in or you will be a bit dehydrated once in a while.

Don't be scared by all the numbers. I provide an early example so that you can easily follow along and use your own numbers to figure out what your body will need. You can also refer to the "Body Weight and Macronutrient Needs" chart (see Figure 3.3) to easily find how much carbohydrate, protein, and fat you should eat based on your current and possibly changing body weight.

Daily Macronutrient and Fluid Needs in the Preparation Cycle

- **Carbohydrate intake should range from 5–7 grams per kilogram of body weight (g/kg) for moderate duration and low intensity training to 7–12 g/kg for moderate to heavy training to 10–12+ g/kg for extreme training (4–6+ hours per day).**

  Nutrition Nibble: I recommend eating at least 6–9 servings of fruits and vegetables during this cycle along with whole grains and starches. This will ensure that you are getting appropriate amounts of vitamins, minerals, and fiber.

- **Protein intake should range from 1.2–1.7 g/kg.**

  Nutrition Nibble: Unless you are a strict vegan and do not eat any animal products, I recommend choosing lean portions of meats and low fat dairy products. You can also get protein from non-animal sources such as beans,

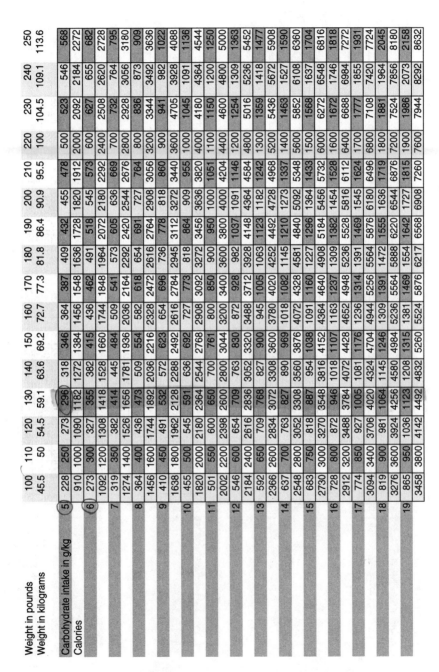

Table: Carbohydrate intake (grams) and Calories by body weight and carbohydrate intake in g/kg.

Carbohydrate intake in g/kg		**Weight in pounds** 100	110	120	130	140	150	160	170	180	190	200	210	220	230	240	250
		Weight in kilograms 45.5	50	54.5	59.1	63.6	69.2	72.7	77.3	81.8	86.4	90.9	95.5	100	104.5	109.1	113.6
5	Carbs (g)	228	250	273	296	318	346	364	387	409	432	455	478	500	523	546	568
5	Calories	910	1000	1090	1182	1272	1384	1456	1548	1636	1728	1820	1912	2000	2092	2184	2272
6	Carbs (g)	273	300	327	355	382	415	436	462	491	518	545	573	600	627	655	682
6	Calories	1092	1200	1308	1418	1528	1660	1744	1848	1964	2072	2180	2292	2400	2508	2620	2728
7	Carbs (g)	319	350	382	414	445	484	509	541	573	605	636	669	700	732	764	795
7	Calories	1274	1400	1526	1656	1781	1936	2036	2164	2292	2420	2544	2676	2800	2928	3056	3180
8	Carbs (g)	364	400	436	473	509	554	582	618	654	691	727	764	800	836	873	909
8	Calories	1456	1600	1744	1892	2036	2216	2328	2472	2616	2764	2908	3056	3200	3344	3492	3636
9	Carbs (g)	410	450	491	532	572	623	654	696	736	778	818	860	900	941	982	1022
9	Calories	1638	1800	1962	2128	2288	2492	2616	2784	2945	3112	3272	3440	3600	3764	3928	4088
10	Carbs (g)	455	500	545	591	636	692	727	773	818	864	909	955	1000	1045	1091	1136
10	Calories	1820	2000	2180	2364	2544	2768	2908	3092	3272	3456	3636	3820	4000	4180	4364	4544
11	Carbs (g)	501	550	600	650	700	761	800	850	900	950	1000	1051	1100	1150	1200	1250
11	Calories	2002	2200	2398	2600	2800	3044	3200	3400	3600	3800	4000	4204	4400	4600	4800	5000
12	Carbs (g)	546	600	654	709	763	830	872	928	982	1037	1091	1146	1200	1254	1309	1363
12	Calories	2184	2400	2616	2836	3052	3320	3488	3712	3928	4148	4364	4584	4800	5016	5236	5452
13	Carbs (g)	592	650	709	768	827	900	945	1005	1063	1123	1182	1242	1300	1359	1418	1477
13	Calories	2366	2600	2834	3072	3308	3600	3780	4020	4252	4492	4728	4968	5200	5436	5672	5908
14	Carbs (g)	637	700	763	827	890	969	1018	1082	1145	1210	1273	1337	1400	1463	1527	1590
14	Calories	2548	2800	3052	3308	3560	3876	4072	4328	4581	4840	5092	5348	5600	5852	6108	6360
15	Carbs (g)	683	750	818	887	954	1038	1091	1160	1227	1296	1364	1433	1500	1568	1637	1704
15	Calories	2730	3000	3270	3548	3816	4152	4364	4640	4908	5184	5456	5732	6000	6272	6548	6816
16	Carbs (g)	728	800	872	946	1018	1107	1163	1237	1309	1382	1454	1528	1600	1672	1746	1818
16	Calories	2912	3200	3488	3784	4072	4428	4652	4948	5236	5528	5816	6112	6400	6688	6984	7272
17	Carbs (g)	774	850	927	1005	1081	1176	1236	1314	1391	1469	1545	1624	1700	1777	1855	1931
17	Calories	3094	3400	3706	4020	4324	4704	4944	5256	5564	5876	6180	6496	6800	7108	7420	7724
18	Carbs (g)	819	900	981	1064	1145	1246	1309	1391	1472	1555	1636	1719	1800	1881	1964	2045
18	Calories	3276	3600	3924	4256	4580	4984	5236	5564	5888	6220	6544	6876	7200	7524	7856	8180
19	Carbs (g)	865	950	1036	1123	1208	1315	1381	1469	1554	1642	1727	1815	1900	1986	2073	2158
19	Calories	3458	3800	4142	4492	4832	5260	5524	5876	6217	6568	6908	7260	7600	7944	8292	8632

Figure 3.3 Body Weight and Macronutrient Needs

BASE - 296g - 355g

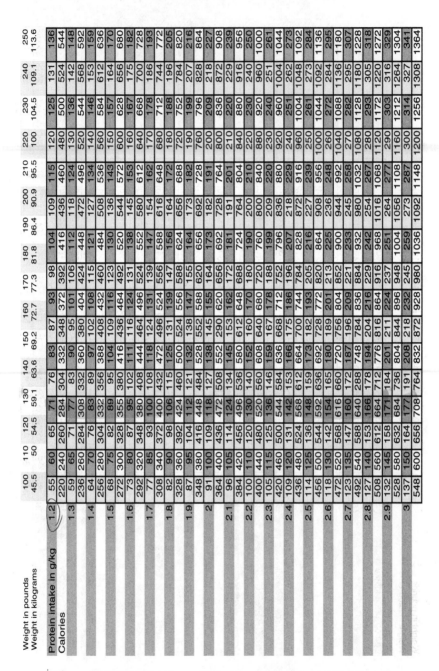

Weight in pounds	100	110	120	130	140	150	160	170	180	190	200	210	220	230	240	250
Weight in kilograms	45.5	50	54.5	59.1	63.6	69.2	72.7	77.3	81.8	86.4	90.9	95.5	100	104.5	109.1	113.6
Protein intake in g/kg																
1.2	55	60	65	71	76	83	87	93	98	104	109	115	120	125	131	136
Calories	220	240	260	284	304	332	348	372	392	416	436	460	480	500	524	544
1.3	59	65	71	77	83	90	95	101	106	112	118	124	130	136	142	148
Calories	236	260	284	308	332	360	380	404	424	448	472	496	520	544	568	592
1.4	64	70	76	83	89	97	102	108	115	121	127	134	140	146	153	159
Calories	256	280	304	332	356	388	408	432	460	484	508	536	560	584	612	636
1.5	68	75	82	89	95	104	109	116	123	130	136	143	150	157	164	170
Calories	272	300	328	355	380	416	436	464	492	520	544	572	600	628	656	680
1.6	73	80	87	95	102	111	116	124	131	138	145	153	160	167	175	182
Calories	292	320	348	380	408	444	464	496	524	552	580	612	640	668	700	728
1.7	77	85	93	100	108	118	124	131	139	147	154	162	170	178	186	193
Calories	308	340	372	400	432	472	496	524	556	588	616	648	680	712	744	772
1.8	82	90	98	106	115	125	131	139	147	156	164	172	180	188	196	205
Calories	328	360	392	424	460	500	524	556	588	624	656	688	720	752	784	820
1.9	87	95	104	112	121	132	138	147	155	164	173	182	190	199	207	216
Calories	348	380	416	448	484	528	552	588	620	656	692	728	760	796	828	864
2	91	100	109	118	127	138	145	155	164	173	182	191	200	209	218	227
Calories	364	400	436	472	508	552	580	620	656	692	728	764	800	836	872	908
2.1	96	105	114	124	134	145	153	162	172	181	191	201	210	220	229	239
Calories	384	420	456	496	536	580	612	648	688	724	764	804	840	880	916	956
2.2	100	110	120	130	140	152	160	170	180	190	200	210	220	230	240	250
Calories	400	440	480	520	560	608	640	680	720	760	800	840	880	920	960	1000
2.3	105	115	125	136	146	159	167	178	188	199	209	220	230	240	251	261
Calories	420	460	500	544	584	636	668	712	752	796	836	880	920	960	1004	1044
2.4	109	120	131	142	153	166	175	186	196	207	218	229	240	251	262	273
Calories	436	480	524	568	612	664	700	744	784	828	872	916	960	1004	1048	1092
2.5	114	125	136	148	159	173	182	193	205	216	227	239	250	261	273	284
Calories	456	500	544	592	636	692	728	772	820	864	908	956	1000	1044	1092	1136
2.6	118	130	142	154	165	180	189	201	213	225	236	248	260	272	284	295
Calories	472	520	568	616	660	720	756	804	852	900	944	992	1040	1088	1136	1180
2.7	123	135	147	160	172	187	196	209	221	233	245	258	270	282	295	307
Calories	492	540	588	640	688	748	784	836	884	932	980	1032	1080	1128	1180	1228
2.8	127	140	153	166	178	194	204	216	229	242	254	267	280	293	305	318
Calories	508	560	612	664	712	776	816	864	916	968	1016	1068	1120	1172	1220	1272
2.9	132	145	158	171	184	201	211	224	237	251	264	277	290	303	316	329
Calories	528	580	632	684	736	804	844	896	948	1004	1056	1108	1160	1212	1264	1304
3	137	150	164	177	191	208	218	232	245	259	273	287	300	314	327	341
Calories	548	600	656	708	764	832	872	928	980	1036	1092	1148	1200	1256	1308	1364

Figure 3.3 Body Weight and Macronutrient Needs (Continued)

(handwritten annotations: "BASE 1.2g/kg", "71g")

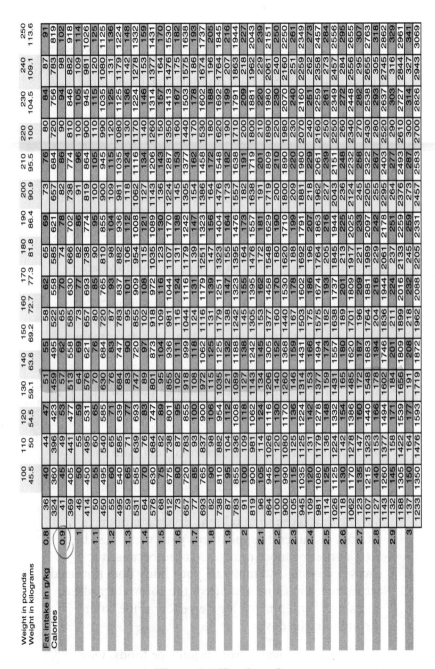

Figure 3.3 (Continued)

nuts, and grains. Another tip is to keep an eye on the amount of iron you eat since some endurance athletes, mostly female, are susceptible to developing iron deficiency anemia during their training year. Choose red meats as a good quality iron source. As a vegetarian option, choose dark green leafy vegetables combined with vitamin C (such as a glass of orange juice).

- **Fat intake should range from 0.8–1.0 g/kg.**

  Nutrition Nibble: With the obvious health concerns surrounding fat intake, it is best to focus on the healthier mono- and polyunsaturated fats. Sources include olives, avocados, fish, nuts, and oils such as canola, flax, and olive. Try to decrease the amount of unhealthy saturated fats such as high-fat animal products. In addition, stay clear of trans fat, which are found in processed foods like cookies, potato chips, and some fast foods. These are fats that are chemically altered and are the worst type of fat that you can eat.

- **Stay hydrated (based on the color of your urine).**

  Nutrition Nibble: Recently, hydration guidelines (the maxim of 8 glasses a day) were challenged because some athletes may require more or less fluid for hydration. The best thing to do is base the amount of fluid you drink on the color of your urine. Aim for straw-colored (pale yellow) urine most times throughout the day. Keep in mind that if you are taking a vitamin or mineral supplement, your urine may be a little darker or more orange-colored because the excess vitamins and minerals your body does not need are excreted in urine and affect the color. Regardless, you should still aim for a pale yellow urine color throughout the day.

  You can get water from liquids or foods. One thing to remember is that you shouldn't wait for your thirst response to signal you to drink more fluids. Once you feel thirsty, you are already dehydrated, so be sure to choose foods that have a high water content, such as fruits and vegetables, and space your drinking throughout the day so you remain hydrated.

See Table 3.1 for a summary of daily needs during this cycle.

Putting it All Together: Daily Nutrition

It is time to put the above recommendations to use and customize a plan for your body. This example will help you set up your daily nutrient requirements, so grab a calculator and use your body weight and training information in place of the example numbers.

This example will use a male endurance athlete, Bobby, who is 5'10" tall and weighs 170 pounds. He wants to remain at his current weight. He trains at a moderate volume (1 hour per weekday and 2.5 hours on each weekend day) and low intensity because he is in the beginning of his preparation cycle. Keep in mind that if you are like most endurance athletes and you train more or less on weekends versus weekdays, your body will need more or less energy on different days, so customize your eating program to meet your training schedule.

This is going to seem like a lot of numbers to work with but it is far less complicated to do this than to set up your physical training and determine when your cycles should be, how long they should last, when you should add speed work, and how much recovery you should take! Remember to refer to the "Body

Table 3.1
Daily Nutrition Needs During the Preparation Mesocycle

Training Cycle	Carbohydrate	Protein	Fat	Fluids
Preparation	5–12+ g/kg	1.2–1.7 g/kg	0.8–1.0 g/kg	enough to produce straw-colored urine

Weight and Macronutrient Needs" chart (Figure 3.3) as a reference so you don't have to calculate all of your numbers. Reading food labels will help you learn the numbers for actual food so I encourage you to glance at a label every so often so you can begin learning what nutrients and what amounts are in the foods you normally eat.

Step 1: Convert pounds to kilograms by dividing pounds by 2.2.

- Bobby weighs 170 pounds.

    170 pounds/2.2 = 77.3 kilograms

Step 2: Figure carbohydrate requirements.

- Since Bobby trains at a moderate volume and low intensity because he is just getting back into training, we will use a carbohydrate recommendation from the lower range of 6 grams per kilogram of body weight.

    6 grams of carbohydrate × 77.3 kilograms of body weight = 464 grams of carbohydrate on weekdays

- Convert grams to calories.

    464 grams of carbohydrate × 4 calories per gram of carbohydrate = 1,856 calories

- Since Bobby trains more on the weekends, we will use a higher carbohydrate recommendation of 10 grams of carbohydrate per kilogram of body weight.

    10 grams of carbohydrate × 77.3 kilograms of body weight = 773 grams of carbohydrate on weekends

- Convert grams to calories.

    773 grams of carbohydrate × 4 calories per gram of carbohydrate = 3,092 calories

Step 3: Figure protein requirements.

- Bobby does low- to moderate-intensity strength training three times per week for 45 minutes per session so his protein requirements are not too high. We will use 1.4 grams of protein per kilogram of body weight as his recommended intake.

  1.4 grams of protein × 77.3 kilograms of body weight = 108 grams of protein on all days

- Convert grams to calories.

  108 grams of protein × 4 calories per gram of protein = 432 calories

Step 4: Figure fat requirements.

- Bobby will follow a fat recommendation of 1.0 gram of fat per kilogram of body weight.

  1.0 gram of fat × 77.3 kilograms of body weight = 77 grams of fat on all days

- Convert grams to calories.

  77 grams of fat × 9 calories per gram of fat = 693 calories

Step 5: Figure total calorie requirements.

- Weekdays:

  1,856 calories from carbohydrate + 432 calories from protein + 693 calories from fat = 2,981 calories per day

- Weekends:

  3,092 calories from carbohydrate + 432 calories from protein + 693 calories from fat = 4,217 calories per day

Summary

On weekdays, Bobby should eat 2,981 calories with 62% of his daily calories consisting of carbohydrates, 15% protein, and 23% fat.

On weekends, because he is training more than he does on weekdays, his requirements are different. He should eat more calories per day (in the form of carbohydrates) to support his increase in training volume. In Bobby's case, he should eat 4,217 calories with 73% of his daily calories from carbohydrates, 10% from protein, and 16% from fat.

Macronutrient and Fluid Timing for Training during the Preparation Cycle

- **Drink 17–20 ounces of fluid 2 hours before training.**

  Nutrition Nibble: Starting a training session already dehydrated is not good for your performance or your health, so plan ahead. Drink enough fluid before training to stay fully hydrated.

- **Drink 7–10 ounces of sports drink 10–20 minutes before training.**

  Nutrition Nibble: It has been my experience that athletes often forget this hydration rule because of so many other things are happening at this time and you are trying to get out the door to train. If you can fill a small flask (like the ones that hold energy gel) with a sports drink and put it in your pocket or somewhere else (by the front door or by your keys) that is easy to get to then you will have it with you and be more likely to drink it than if you have to search for it. Minimize your distractions and worries before an intense workout and carry a sports drink with you to avoid frantically searching for it at the last minute.

gatrade

powerbar

- **Consume 30–60 grams of carbohydrate per hour of training.**

  Nutrition Nibble: Depending on your digestive system, you can choose a solid or liquid form of carbohydrate. Remember that during moderate-intensity exercise, blood flow in the gut is moderate, which means you should be able to choose easily digestible carbohydrates such as energy bars and bagels, but during higher intensity exercise, blood flow in the gut is lower, which means you should consume more liquids and gels since your digestive system will not be able to efficiently break down the solid foods. Keep in mind that many sports bars have some fiber in them, which means the possibility of more frequent bathroom breaks. Avoid these or plan accordingly!

- **Drink 7–10 ounces of fluid every 15–20 minutes during training.**

  Nutrition Nibble: It is always a good idea to choose a sports drink that contains sodium to replace lost electrolytes and prevent muscle cramping and hyponatremia. An easy way to remember to stay hydrated is to set your watch interval to go off every 15–20 minutes to remind you to drink. I highly recommend a sports drink with at least 110–200 milligrams of sodium per 8 ounces for training that will last longer than 30 minutes. The body is in need of carbohydrates after this time and is losing both water and sodium through sweat. However, you may find that you need to begin hydrating sooner. There is nothing magic about these numbers. What is important is that you prevent dehydration, so if you need to start drinking 5 minutes into your exercise, then please do so!

  If you find yourself not wanting to follow this guideline during training because it is too difficult to carry that much fluid, you can either hide extra water bottles on your training course, learn gas stations that you can stop at to re-hydrate, or have a friend or family member meet you at certain times and locations during your training.

- **Drink 20–24 ounces of fluid for every pound of body weight lost after training.**

  Nutrition Nibble: A good practice to get into is to weigh yourself before you go out for a longer training session and weigh yourself when you get back. This will make it much easier for you to figure out how much fluid you should drink to re-hydrate yourself. Remember that sodium helps facilitate glucose (sugar) getting into your cells to replenish the glucose that you used during training so choose a sports drink with sodium.

- **After training within the first 30 minutes, eat 1.0–1.2 grams of carbohydrate per kilogram of body weight. In addition, eat 6–20 grams of protein if the training session is >90 minutes.**

  Nutrition Nibble: Most research supports that there will not be a compromise in muscle glycogen delivery when protein is consumed after exercise and protein may speed muscle tissue repair and provide important nutrients for the immune system. If your training is less than 90 minutes, just focus on eating carbohydrates.

- **Following the training session, eat another 1.0–1.2 grams of carbohydrate per kilogram of body weight 2 hours after the initial carbohydrate feeding.**

  Nutrition Nibble: It is best to eat this in the form of a regular well-balanced meal. Good choices are a turkey sandwich without mayonnaise, pizza with minimal cheese, or a nonfat milk-based fruit smoothie.

See Table 3.2 for a summary of training needs during this cycle.

Putting it All Together: Recovery Nutrition

Here is an example to help you develop a nutrition recovery plan to use after training during the preparation mesocycle. We will use the same athlete that we used earlier: Bobby, a male endurance athlete who is 5'10" tall and weighs 170 pounds.

Step 1: Figure carbohydrate requirements.

- We will use the upper recommendation of 1.2 grams of carbohydrate per kilogram of body weight. (Remember to adjust according to your own training level.)

  1.2 grams of carbohydrate × 77.3 kilograms of body weight = 93 grams

- Convert grams to calories.

  93 grams of carbohydrate × 4 calories per gram of carbohydrate = 372 calories

Table 3.2
Training Needs during the Preparation Mesocycle

Nutrient	Pre-training	During training	Post-training
Fluid	17–20 oz. at 2 hours 7–10 ounces at 10–20 minutes	7–10 oz. every 15–20 minutes, include sodium	20–24 oz. for every pound of weight lost, include sodium
Carbohydrate	X Not always needed during the first part of this cycle	30–60 grams (120–240 calories) per hour	1.0–1.2 g/kg in first 30 minutes and then at 2-hour intervals
Protein	X	X	6–20 grams in first 30 minutes and then a mixed meal 2 hours later
Fat	X	X	minimal after 2–4 hours

Step 2: Figure protein requirements if the training session is longer than 90 minutes.

- We will use 10 grams of protein in this example.

    10 grams of protein × 4 calories per gram of
    protein = 40 calories

Step 3: Repeat step 1 and eat the same amount of carbohydrates (372 calories) 2 hours after the initial feeding.

Summary

Bobby will eat a total of 412 calories soon after finishing his training session. Most athletes find it easiest to consume these calories in a liquid form, so commercial sports drinks or home-made nonfat milk-based fruit smoothies are good choices.

General and Specific Eating Guidelines for the Preparation Cycle

- **Eat a minimum of 6–9 servings of fruits and vegetables per day to make sure you get enough vitamins, minerals, and phytochemicals.**

    Nutrition Nibble: I know that this may seem difficult but remember that portion sizes are relatively small for fruits and vegetables. Refer to Chapter 2 for more information about serving sizes.

    Phytochemicals are beneficial chemical compounds found in plants that may help prevent cancer and heart disease by acting as antioxidants. Common plant sources of phytochemicals include citrus fruits, potatoes, onions, garlic, soy, and dark green leafy vegetables

- **Choose high-fiber foods.**

    Nutrition Nibble: Some fiber promotes regularity and other types help to lower cholesterol levels. While regularity may not seem important during this cycle, think about the consequences of ignoring this issue. Constipation can cause severe bowel distress and can lead to stomachaches, which may lead to decreased training sessions because of feeling ill. Hemorrhoids could be even worse. Be sure to eat your fiber!

Insoluble fiber (roughage) is made up of the woody or structural parts of plants and is found in some fruits and vegetables, whole grains, beans, and wheat bran. This type of fiber tends to speed the passage of material through the digestive tract. It is helpful in preventing and treating constipation. Soluble fiber, beneficial for reducing cholesterol levels, dissolves and thickens in water to form gels; it is found in foods such as beans, oatmeal, barley, oat bran, broccoli, raw carrots, cabbage, peaches, plums, bananas, and citrus fruits.

- **Try new foods and experiment.**

Nutrition Nibble: Food is essential to life but it should be fun also. Have fun with your eating program and mix it up a little by trying new ethnic foods, different food preparation methods, and exotic fruits and vegetables. Experimentation may be easiest during the preparation and transition cycles; you don't want to experiment right before your most important race.

- **Experiment with different energy bars, gels, and sports drinks during this cycle in order to learn which products agree with your body.**

Nutrition Nibble: There are many nutrition bars, gels, and drinks on the market that claim to provide the same benefits. Some of them use different sugars in different amounts. It is up to you to find the combination of ingredients that works best for your specific needs. Also, remember to avoid sports drinks that have a carbohydrate concentration greater than 8%. This slows down the time it takes to get it out of your stomach.

- **Find out what nutritional products will be used at your races in the upcoming season and try them in training.**

  Nutrition Nibble: Race directors usually depend on sponsorship for this and rarely get to choose which products that they will use. If they do not list the products in their race information, contact them directly and ask them. The worst thing you can do is train with products that work well for your body during training and then use other products that you have not tried during your race. You are just asking for digestive problems! If you find that you cannot use the products that will be at your race, there are ways of carrying most of your fluid and food. There are specific belts and packs that you can wear in which you can store almost all of your drinks, bars, and gels.

- **Don't forget about the environment.**

  Nutrition Nibble: If it is cold it is still necessary to drink. Cold weather doesn't change the amount of sweat glands that your body has. I know it may be difficult to hydrate on a consistent basis because of cold weather and layers of clothes that you may be wearing but remember you can always stop for a few seconds to take a drink!

- **Don't get in the rut of eating the same thing everyday.**

  Nutrition Nibble: Rotate through different foods and menus in order to get more overall variety and balance in your eating plan. Did you know that an average American only eats 50 different foods compared to people in other societies who eat well over 100 different foods? The more variety you have in your eat-

ing program, the better the balance of nutrients you
will get and the healthier you will be.

The Competition Mesocycle (aka the Intensity or Build Cycle) *B.*

It is time to turn up the intensity! Now you will begin to
improve your functional and sport-specific strength and speed.
Intensity will be increasing, while your volume will be staying
fairly moderate in order to allow for quality strength and speed
work with ample recovery time afterwards. Your physiological
goals include improving your body's ability to handle and clear
lactate, which in turn will allow you to race stronger and faster.
During this mesocycle, you will be burning a large amount of
calories through training, so don't try to actively lose weight. If
you do, the quality of your training will suffer and you will not
be developing your lactate-clearing abilities the best you can.

The biggest mistake that you can make during this mesocycle
is to not eat. Your body requires carbohydrates, protein, and fat
continually for energy and recovery, so set your nutrition plan
based on your training duration and intensity. Since this mesocycle is divided into a pre-race phase and a race phase, the information in this section is also divided accordingly.

The Pre-race Cycle

Daily Macronutrient and Fluid Needs in the Pre-race Cycle

- **Carbohydrate intake should range from 7–13 g/kg.**

  Nutrition Nibble: This is a similar range as for your
  preparation cycle but because you will most likely
  be doing at least two speed sessions of some type
  each week, you should choose the higher end of the
  recommended range of carbohydrates per kilogram

of body weight on these days. Don't forget that you will be burning more calories and your body will need more energy from carbohydrates to make it through your speed sessions.

- **Protein intake should range from 1.4–2.0 g/kg.**

  Nutrition Nibble: This is a little higher recommendation than I made for you during your preparation cycle due to the higher stress you place on your muscles during more intense speed training sessions and strength training.

- **Fat intake should range from 0.8–3.0 g/kg.**

  Nutrition Nibble: Be sure to focus on eating healthy fats during this time. Don't allow your mind to play tricks on you and justify reaching for the chips or cookies with unhealthy fats. Remember, sports nutrition is just as much about health as it is about performance.

- **Fluid guidelines remain the same as described in the preparation period.**

  Nutrition Nibble: Keep your environment in mind. Some athletes will begin their pre-race cycle when the weather is getting warmer. Heat increases the body's fluid requirements. Be sure to drink more throughout the day and monitor the color of your urine.

Daily nutrition needs for this cycle are summed up in Table 3.3.

Macronutrient and Fluid Timing for Training during the Pre-Race Cycle

- **Drink 17–20 ounces of fluid 2 hours before training.**

- **Drink 7–10 ounces of sports drink 10–20 minutes before training.**

- Consume 30–60 grams of carbohydrate per hour of training.

  Nutrition Nibble: If you are doing speed intervals, it will be difficult to eat during them. If you can eat a gel or two per hour, then do so, but if the workout intensity is too high for you to think about eating anything, just choose a sports drink with carbohydrates and sodium (see next recommendation).

- Drink 7–10 ounces of fluid every 15–20 minutes during training.

- Drink 20–24 ounces of fluid for every pound of body weight lost after training.

  Nutrition Nibble: It is extremely important to weigh yourself before and after speed interval sessions since you will typically lose more weight during these due to the increase in calories burned. You will also want to make sure that you are fully re-hydrated for the next day of training in case you have speed sessions close to one another (this is not recommended but I have seen athletes do this).

- Within 30 minutes after training, eat 1.0–1.2 grams of carbohydrate per kilogram of body weight. In addition, eat 6–20 grams of protein if the training session is >90 minutes.

Table 3.3
Daily Nutrition Needs during the Pre-race Cycle

Training Cycle	Carbohydrate	Protein	Fat	Fluids
Pre-race	7–13 g/kg	1.4–2.0 g/kg	0.8–2.0 g/kg	enough to produce straw-colored urine

- Eat 1.0–1.2 grams of carbohydrate per kilogram of body weight 2 hours after the initial carbohydrate feeding following the training session.

See Table 3.4 for a summary of training needs during this cycle.

General and Specific Eating Guidelines for the Pre-race Cycle

- Stick with the energy bars, gels, and sports drinks that worked well for you in the preparation cycle.

  Nutrition Nibble: Try to be consistent from here on out with the energy bars, gels, and sports drinks that you use. You don't want to change your choices midseason and risk stomach problems during a race.

Table 3.4
Training Needs during the Pre-race cycle

Nutrient	Pre-training	During training	Post-training
Fluid	17–20 oz. at 2 hours 7–10 ounces at 10–20 minutes	7–10 oz. every 15–20 minutes, include sodium	20–24 oz. for every pound of weight lost, include sodium
Carbohydrate	1–4 g/kg at 1–4 hours	30–60 grams (120–240 calories) per hour	1.0–1.2 g/kg in first 30 minutes and then at 2-hour intervals
Protein	X	Questionable	6–20 grams in first 30 minutes and then a mixed meal 2 hours later
Fat	X	X	minimal at 2–4 hours

- **Eat often. Snacking is beneficial in this cycle.**

  Nutrition Nibble: Because you are training at a higher intensity, your body will need calories more often throughout the day. Be sure to carry snacks such as energy bars, fruit, whole wheat crackers, or yogurt wherever you go so you have some type of nutritious food with you at all times.

- **Increase sodium intake if you are not salt-sensitive and do not have high blood pressure.**

  Nutrition Nibble: Depending on the race environmental conditions and the distance, additional dietary sodium may be of benefit. Just add a few sprinkles of salt to most of your daily meals. Salt tablets are extremely popular and if you think you may use these in races, experiment with the different brands and amounts of sodium found in each during this cycle. Try salt tablets in a longer, race-simulation workout to closely mimic race conditions. It is always best to try your race nutrition plan during a race-simulation workout rather than during a lower intensity workout since the body processes food and drink differently at low and high levels of intensity.

- **Don't skimp on the calories, but don't think that you can eat everything and anything you want just because you are training hard.**

  Nutrition Nibble: Because intensity is high, energy expenditure will also be high. The amount of food you eat must be adequate to replace the calories that you burn in training without experiencing significant, long-term weight loss. You will lose a couple of pounds after training sessions but your re-hydration and recovery nutrition should prevent this short-term weight loss from developing into chronic weight loss.

The Race Cycle

Your race season should have two goals: (1) improvement in race performance, and (2) proper recovery to improve your perform-ance in your next race. This cycle will still include a fairly high level of intensity but a significant reduction in volume since you are racing. Your physiological goals are to reap the benefits of your well-planned training in the previous two periodization cycles (the preparation mesocycle and the pre-race portion of the competition mesocycle) and race as hard and fast as you can. The distances that you compete in will usually dictate at what inten-sity you will race but you are normally pushing your lactate threshold and oftentimes racing at or above it for a good portion of your races. Because of the increased physiological demands that this cycle puts on your body, your nutrition leading up to, right before, during, and after a race are extremely important, especially if you will be racing at least twice per month.

There is a very large range of nutrient needs during this cycle. The reason for this is that endurance athletes compete in such a wide variety of events, from sprint triathlons to the Race Across America cycling event to adventure races. I provide you the broad range so that you have a starting place to begin with your nutrition plan.

In general, if your race will take you less than 5 hours, you can follow the nutrition periodization guidelines found in the pre-race cycle. If your race will take from 5–12 hours, you should start with the middle range of the nutrient needs presented next, and if your race will last longer than 12 hours, you should start with the higher range of the nutrient needs listed. Based on your previous training cycle, you should have a very good idea of how much your body needs long before you enter this competitive cycle.

Daily Macronutrient and Fluid Needs in the Race Cycle

- **Carbohydrate intake should range from 7–19 g/kg.**

  Nutrition Nibble: If you will be racing at a fairly high intensity (greater than 75% of your maximum heart rate or VO_2 max), then carbohydrate will be the main source of energy for your body and you should focus on consuming more carbohydrates than protein and fat. If you can constantly eat carbohydrates, your need for protein and fat will be minimal unless you are competing in multi-day races.

- **Protein intake should range from 1.2–2.0 g/kg.**

  Nutrition Nibble: You only need protein if your race will last longer than 90 minutes. In that case, you should choose the lower edge of this range, unless you are doing a multi-day race, to avoid any possible stomach and digestive problems. Increase your protein intake, up to 2.0 g/kg of protein, when you are in a heavy training cycle.

- **Fat intake should be 0.8–3.0 g/kg.**

  Nutrition Nibble: If you are not doing a multi-day race, you do not need to worry about eating fat during your race. It will just cause digestive and carbohydrate absorption problems.

- **Increase fluid intake.**

  Nutrition Nibble: Because you will be losing much more water and electrolytes due to the higher intensity at which you will be racing, it is recommended to slightly increase the amount of fluid you drink during the day. Remember, being aware of your urine color is the best way to monitor your hydration status.

See Table 3.5 for a summary of your daily nutrition needs during this cycle.

Macronutrient and Fluid Timing for Racing during the Race Cycle

- **Consume 1–4 grams of carbohydrate per kilogram of body weight 1–4 hours before the race.**

  Nutrition Nibble: When you first wake up in the morning, you are in a fasted state because your body is using your stored glucose while you sleep. By eating 1–4 hours before your race, you are topping off your "gas tank", making sure that your stored energy levels are full. Keep in mind that this usually means waking up pretty early on race day. You may have to get up as early as 2:00 or 3:00 in the morning but you can go back to sleep after eating if possible. It is crucial to eat this amount before the start of your race, so set a couple of alarms so you do not forget to eat!

- **Drink 17–20 ounces of fluid 2 hours before your race.**

- **Drink 7–10 ounces of sports drink 10–20 minutes before your race.**

Table 3.5
Daily Nutrition Needs During the Race Cycle

Training Cycle	Carbohydrate	Protein	Fat	Fluids
Competition	7–19 g/kg	1.2–2.0 g/kg	0.8–3.0 g/kg	enough to produce pale or straw-colored urine

- **Consume 30–100 grams of carbohydrate per hour during your race.**

  Nutrition Nibble: I mentioned earlier that the body of the average person can absorb about 1 gram of carbohydrate per minute (60 grams per hour). It has been my experience that some athletes can absorb more carbohydrates without problems, toward the upper limit of 100 grams per hour (or 1.7 grams per minute), and sometimes even more. These athletes are few and far between but you should use this upper limit to gauge your specific nutrition needs. In races that will take longer than 24 hours or multi-day races, you may need to eat up to that many carbohydrates per hour to simply stay in energy balance. The brain gets about 95% of its energy from glucose (carbohydrates) so you may need to eat a large amount of carbohydrates to sustain your mental focus as well.

  The important thing to remember is that you are different from all of your competitors and training partners and what works for them will not necessarily work for you. Start conservatively, look at what worked for you in your previous periodization cycles, and adapt your nutrition needs to the race distance and environment in which you will be competing.

- **Drink 7–10 ounces of fluid every 15–20 minutes during your race.**

  Nutrition Nibble: Using a sports drink that contains adequate carbohydrates and sodium is always preferred during races no matter the distance.

- **After your race, drink 20–24 ounces of fluid for every pound of body weight lost.**

  Nutrition Nibble: Remember, adding sodium to the fluid, as a sports drink does, helps the carbohydrate and fluid get into your body's cells better. That's why a sports drink is the best choice for post-race fluid recovery needs.

- **Within the first 30 minutes after your race, eat 1.0–1.2 grams of carbohydrate per kilogram of body weight. In addition, eat 6–20 grams of protein if your race was >90 minutes.**

- **Two hours after the initial carbohydrate feeding following your race, eat 1.0–1.2 grams of carbohydrate per kilogram of body weight.**

See Table 3.6 for a summary of your training needs during this cycle.

Carbohydrate Loading

Carbohydrate loading has been proven to be of great benefit to the endurance athlete in races longer than 2 hours. There are many carbohydrate loading protocols out there but I have chosen the most popular and the simplest one to follow. Be sure to begin your carbohydrate loading regimen at least one week before your race. During this time, your protein and fat intake should stay the same as they have been during your training except for during the last 2–3 days. During these days, decrease the amount of protein and fat that you eat so that you can ensure that adequate digestion takes place. Remember, it takes 48–72 hours for food to leave our bodies after we place it in our mouth.

Truth be told, you will gain weight during this carbohydrate loading phase. A normal weight gain for most athletes is about 2–3 pounds but it will be lost quickly once exercise begins. Do not be alarmed as this is actually very beneficial to you. Because water is bound to carbohydrates in a 3:1 ratio of water to carbohydrates, extra water is stored in your body and in your cells. While it does increase body weight, it also tops off your fluid "gas tank", which is a very good thing. Having a "full tank"

Table 3.6
Training Needs during the Race Cycle

Nutrient	Pre-race	During the race	Post-race
Fluid	17–20 oz. at 2 hours 7–10 ounces at 10–20 minutes	7–10 oz. every 15–20 minutes, include sodium	20–24 oz. for every pound of weight lost, include sodium
Carbohydrate	1–4 g/kg at 1–4 hours	30–100 grams (120–400 calories) per hour	1.0–1.2 g/kg in first 30 minutes and then at 2 hour intervals
Protein	X	Questionable	6–20 grams in first 30 minutes and then a mixed meal 2 hours later
Fat	X	X	minimal at 2–4 hours

before you compete is the goal so that you do not get too dehydrated during your race.

Carbohydrate loading regimen

- Consume at least 5 grams of carbohydrate per kilogram of body weight per day for the 4–7 days before the race.
- Consume 10 grams of carbohydrate per kilogram of body weight per day for the 1–3 days before the race. Remember to have your large carbohydrate meal two nights before the race and go lighter the night before the race.

This carbohydrate loading protocol has been proven to be effective for most endurance athletes. However, you may have to alter the amount of carbohydrates that you load depending on your current carbohydrate consumption and the duration of your race. For example, if you have been eating 7 grams of carbohydrate per kilogram of body weight during the pre-race cycle, you should not decrease this amount to 5 grams of carbohydrate per kilogram of body weight. If you were eating at the upper range, start the carbohydrate loading at the amount of carbohydrates you are currently eating and increase them to around 10 grams of carbohydrate per kilogram of body weight.

Example:

Back to our friend Bobby, our example of a male endurance athlete who is 5'10" tall and weighs 170 pounds. His race will take him approximately 4 hours to finish and is on a Sunday. Here we'll figure out Bobby's carbohydrate needs for the Sunday, Monday, Tuesday, and Wednesday before his race.

Step 1: Convert pounds to kilograms by dividing pounds by 2.2.

170 pounds/2.2 = 77.3 kilograms

Step 2: Figure carbohydrate loading requirements.

- The carbohydrate requirement for the loading regimen starts at 5 grams of carbohydrate per kilogram of body weight for these 4–7 days before Bobby's race.

  5 grams of carbohydrate × 77.3 kilograms = 387 grams of carbohydrate

- Convert grams to calories.

  387 grams of carbohydrate × 4 calories per gram of carbohydrate = 1,548 calories

Step 3: Figure protein requirements.

- The protein requirement will be the same as before. We will use 1.4 grams of protein per kilogram of body weight.

  1.4 grams of protein × 77.3 kilograms of body weight = 108 grams of protein

- Convert grams to calories.

    108 grams of protein × 4 calories per gram of protein = 432 calories

Step 4: Figure fat requirements.

- Bobby will follow normal recommendations of 1.0 gram of fat per kilogram of body weight.

    1.0 gram of fat × 77.3 kilograms of body weight = 77 grams of fat

Convert grams to calories.

    77 grams of fat × 9 calories per gram of fat = 693 calories

Step 5: Figure minimum total calorie requirements.

- This is a minimum.

    1,548 calories from carbohydrate + 432 calories from protein + 693 calories from fat = 2,673 calories per day

Now we will figure carbohydrate needs for the Thursday and Friday before his race.

Step 1: Convert pounds to kilograms by dividing pounds by 2.2.

    170 pounds/2.2 = 77.3 kilograms

Step 2: Figure carbohydrate loading requirements.

- The carbohydrate requirement for the two days before the race is 10 grams of carbohydrate per kilogram of body weight.

    10 grams of carbohydrate × 77.3 kilograms = 773 grams of carbohydrate

- Convert grams to calories.

    773 grams of carbohydrate × 4 calories per gram of carbohydrate = 3,092 calories

Step 3: Figure protein requirements.

- We will use 1.2 grams of protein per kilogram of body weight now because it is just a few days before his competition.

  1.2 grams of protein × 77.3 kilograms of body weight = 93 grams of protein

- Convert grams to calories.

  93 grams of protein × 4 calories per gram of protein = 372 calories

Step 4: Figure fat requirements.

- Bobby will eat 0.8 grams of fat per kilogram of body weight now.

  0.8 gram of fat × 77.3 kilograms of body weight = 62 grams of fat

- Convert grams to calories:

  62 grams of fat × 9 calories per gram of fat = 558 calories

Step 5: Figure total calorie requirements.

  3,092 calories from carbohydrate + 372 calories from protein + 558 calories from fat = 4,022 calories per day.

- This is more than 1,000 calories more than the first four days of his carbohydrate loading and is meant to top off his stored glycogen tank so that he is ready to go on race day.

Remember, eat your largest meal two nights before your race. You should still eat 10 grams of carbohydrate per kilogram the day before the race, but space it into 7–9 small meals or snacks so you do not eat one large meal. But, again, customize this to your body and your specific needs.

General and Specific Eating Guidelines for the Race Cycle

- **Increase fluid intake to ensure adequate hydration throughout the day.**

  Nutrition Nibble: Keep using your urine color as a marker of hydration status with pale yellow or clear being the goal.

- **Add extra salt to the foods you normally eat if the competition will last longer than 8 hours OR if you know you are a heavy and salty sweater, no matter the distance.**

  Nutrition Nibble: Begin about two weeks before your race and be generous with the salt shaker. Try to add about one teaspoon of extra salt per day (This is only assuming you have no pre-existing health conditions that could be affected by an increased sodium intake).

- **Use the energy bars, gels, and sports drinks that have worked during previous training cycles.**

  Nutrition Nibble: You have heard it everywhere before and I will repeat it again because it is just as true for your nutrition plan: don't try anything new before a race.

- **Develop a pre-race eating routine with specific foods and beverages and specific timing of foods.**

  Nutrition Nibble: Quite honestly, planning and "researching" for this should begin in your preparation, or base, cycle. There are many foods and combinations of foods that you will go through trying to determine what works best for you. The worst routine is no routine at all. Do not get caught close to your race without knowing which eating routine works for you. Experiment early on and keep a written nutrition log regarding what you ate, how much, and at what times so you have something to reference before your race.

- **Slowly increase the amount of sodium an additional amount 3 days before the race if you are a heavy and salty sweater.**

  Nutrition Nibble: Carrying those salt packets from cafeterias is a great way to ensure that you will have enough sodium throughout the day. Remember though, it is best to add this to food, not to eat it straight from the packet. If you do eat it from the packet (or take salt tablets), be sure to have ample water with you to chase it down.

- **Slowly decrease the amount of fiber eaten in the normal diet to prepare for the race day and minimize the chances of frequent bowel movements during the race.**

  Nutrition Nibble: Follow a low-fiber diet starting 2–3 days before the race. Decrease the amount of fruits, vegetables, whole grains, and energy bars that you eat. Good things to eat include fruit and vegetable juices, white bread, and canned goods. I know these suggestions are not high on the healthy meter but you will eat them only for a very short time. It won't be long enough to develop into a habit or have adverse health consequences. However, it is extremely important for you to try this in training first as a rapid switch to a low-fiber diet could result in constipation or hemorrhoids. I have said it before and will say it again: customize this to your body. A lower-fiber diet may be right for you and it may not be. You know your body better than anyone.

- **Decrease use of hot spices to prevent heartburn or GI distress 2–3 days before the race.**

  Nutrition Nibble: Most races have carbohydrate loading dinners that include pasta. Try to limit the meatballs and red pepper that you may put on your pasta. Avoiding any spice that may cause heartburn during this time is highly recommended. Since the chances are that you will be eating out sometime during your race week, be sure to ask your server at the restaurant exactly how the food is prepared.

- **Eat the carbohydrate-loading meal two nights before the race instead of the night before.**

  Nutrition Nibble: More and more races are catching onto this but the majority of races that have been around for a long time still offer the traditional night-before carbohydrate-loading dinner. This is not a good idea. Your body needs adequate time (at least 24–72 hours) to promote adequate digestion of nutrients through the stomach and small intestine so they are absorbed into the bloodstream and stored in the body, ready for use in the race.

  In addition, your anxiety level will most likely be pretty high the day before your race and you won't be able to eat much on race day, so smaller, frequent meals are best on these two days.

- **Graze the day before the race on high-carbohydrate, high-sodium, low-fiber snacks to prevent blood sugar levels from dropping.**

  Nutrition Nibble: One way to do this is to carry a fanny pack or backpack that will hold at least two water bottles wherever you go the day before a race. Fill the water bottles with sports drink and try to finish two of them each hour. Some companies make higher-carbohydrate drinks with no protein, fat, or sodium. These may be good choices if your regular sports drink doesn't provide many calories.

- **Eat breakfast.**

  Nutrition Nibble: By eating a carbohydrate-rich breakfast, you will ensure that your internal gas tank is full and you are ready to race.

- **Don't try anything new right before a race, especially on the day of competition.**

  Nutrition Nibble: Honestly, if you do, you deserve the consequences of your actions!

- **Don't drink too much water.**

  Nutrition Nibble: Hyponatremia, low amounts of sodium in the body, can develop as a result of consuming too much water because it displaces extracellular sodium. Choose a sports drink during all races. It provides water, carbohydrates, and sodium!

Case Study for Competitive Cycle Nutrition

Below is a case study of an athlete that I helped to prepare for his eighth Ironman race. This will help you visualize what I have been stating in words and help you apply it to your specific race nutrition plan.

Mark came to me in August of 2002 and asked me to help him plan his nutrition leading up to and through Ironman New Zealand, which was held in March of 2003. Mark is a recreational athlete. He has completed seven Ironman races and experienced GI distress in all of them. He weighs 155 pounds and is 5'10" tall. His goals were to finish Ironman New Zealand without GI distress and in under 12 hours, which would be a new personal record for him. Because Mark wanted to break his previous personal record, we decided that his race intensity would be close to 80% of his maximum heart rate for the duration of the race. Carbohydrate intake and timing would be crucial to his success. It is important to note here that Mark's training supported his ability to race this Ironman at 80% of his maximum heart rate; this is not the typical race intensity for an Ironman race.

Based on Mark's goal times for each discipline, we estimated his caloric expenditure to be approximately 650 calories during the swim, 5,000 calories during the bike, and 3,500 calories during the run for a total caloric expenditure of 9,150 calories (not including his time in transitions one and two, which is usually fairly minimal, or would be for Mark since he was racing for time).

Mark likely has a glycogen storage capacity of around 1,800 calories, which is typical for a male athlete his size. Given this, he will diminish his internal stores in the first hour of the bike leg. Mark needs 9,150 calories during his Ironman and will exhaust his 1,800 stored glycogen calories by the end of the second hour of the competition. This leaves 10 hours for him to take in the calories he needs to avoid a negative energy balance that may affect his performance. Since he needs to consume 7,350 calories during the last 10 hours of the Ironman, this means Mark must get 735 calories per hour. This isn't too realistic from a physiological standpoint and the logistics of an Ironman make trying to consume that many calories while competing almost impossible. Since we could not get him all 7,350 calories during the competition, our plan was to have Mark replenish his energy stores to his body's upper limit and try to prevent him from becoming undernourished.

The goals we set for Mark's nutrition plan were the following:

1. Proper pre-race nutrition and carbohydrate loading to ensure that his muscle and liver glycogen stores were at their fullest.
2. Adequate fluid and electrolyte intake to delay dehydration.
3. Maximum calorie intake per hour during the race that could be supported by Mark's body to deliver the necessary energy needed for muscular contraction and mental acuity.
4. Proper nutrition after the race to enhance recovery.

Mark began his nutrition taper 2 weeks prior to race day. I provided him with guidelines identical to those listed previously in the race periodization cycle.

Keep in mind that a physical taper for an Ironman race begins 3–5 weeks prior to the race and training volume will be less and, therefore, energy expenditure will be decreased relative to the larger-volume training cycles. A general rule is to decrease volume 15–25% per week, which means caloric intake should also be reduced until the carbohydrate-loading phase.

Race-day nutrition is highly individualized and oftentimes the general rule of thumb is, "If it tastes OK in training, chances are it won't work in a race. If it tastes great in training, it might work in a race." Because racing situations greatly magnify and change the taste of all food and drink, it is important to remember that the best source of calories for an Ironman is the one that the athlete can get down and keep down.

Many options exist for athletes to eat during an Ironman—some of the less traditional items that I have seen used have included peanut butter crackers, fig bars, peanut butter and jelly sandwiches, and candy bars. You have to eat what works for you. The key to successful race-day nutrition is to find foods, gels, liquids, or a combination of all these that's proven effective for you in race-simulation training. During race-simulation training the athlete's Ironman pace should be mimicked in order to see what the GI response to certain foods will be. Often athletes try several nutrition options during lower-intensity training when digestion is not impaired because there is more blood flow centrally to facilitate the digestive process. This will not indicate what you will tolerate under race conditions.

On race morning, Mark needed to eat something to "top off" his glycogen stores. I advised Mark to eat about 1–4 grams of carbohydrate per kilogram of body weight 1–4 hours before the start of the race and drink 17–20 ounces of sports drink during this time. I also recommended that he drink 7–10 ounces of a sports drink about 10–20 minutes prior to the start.

In general, Ironman athletes should consume 60–100 grams of carbohydrate per hour and 28–40 ounces of fluid per hour. Mark and I experimented with various calorie levels, foods, and fluids during his race-simulation training days and found that Mark's body could manage 300 calories per hour from gel and 150 calories per hour from sports drink. He could obtain none of his calories from solid food since it caused severe intestinal cramping with him. To consume this number of calories, he had to eat three energy gels and drink one full bottle of sports drink per hour. In addition, Mark needed to consume 12–16 ounces of water per hour.

Because hyponatremia has increased in prevalence among Ironman athletes, Mark and I also set sodium-intake guidelines for his race. At first during training, I instructed Mark to consume his sodium via his sports drink, Gatorade (110 milligrams of sodium per 8 ounce serving) so we could use that as a baseline to see if any additional sodium was required by his body. Mark drank 44 ounces of Gatorade per hour in training (605 mg sodium/hour). We realized that Mark was a heavy sweater and required more sodium to prevent cramps and hyponatremia. Through a bit of trial and error, we came to the conclusion that Mark would need an additional 350 mg of sodium per hour of cycling to prevent cramping, so he was instructed to follow his normal Gatorade schedule but to also add two salt tablets per hour (each salt tablet had 180 mg sodium).

Because Mark would be in the water for just over 1 hour, it was important for him to begin his nutrition plan immediately upon getting on his bike. Mark's plan was to drink 12 ounces of sports drink within the first mile of the bike ride. Keep in mind that this was a lake swim and drinking a sports drink shortly after exiting the water was palatable. For ocean swims in salt water, I first recommend flushing the salt from the mouth with water, then following with a sports drink.

When gut blood flow is moderate (during moderate-intensity exercise), athletes can consume easily digestible carbohydrates such as sports bars and bagels, but when gut blood flow is low (during higher-intensity exercise), athletes should consume more liquids and gels to promote rapid gastric emptying and intestinal absorption. We knew that Mark would be racing this Ironman at a higher intensity, which would decrease gut blood flow so his nutrition plan included gels and liquids throughout his entire race.

In Mark's previous Ironman races, he had experienced severe GI distress and vomiting during the run. By revisiting the nutrition strategies he used in past races and experimenting in training, we came to realize that he had eaten too many calories per hour from solid foods and not enough sodium in previous Ironman races. To avoid repeating past mistakes, we were conservative with his nutrition during the run. Our plan was to have Mark drink 4 ounces of Gatorade at every aid station beginning with mile 3 and ending at mile 25, for a total of 88 ounces of sports drink and 1,210 mg of sodium. Knowing that the Gatorade provided at aid stations is generally diluted or too sweet and that Mark is a heavy sweater, our plan advised him to consume an additional 180 mg of sodium per hour in salt tablet form and follow it with 4 ounces of water during the run. He was also to eat one energy gel every 30 minutes with 4 ounces of water. This would provide him with approximately 200 calories per hour.

Mark's nutrition plan for his Ironman would result in him consuming 3,900 calories. This is less than half of what we predicted he would expend (9,150 calories). Mark went into Ironman New Zealand physically, mentally, and nutritionally prepared. While he missed achieving a new PR by only 22 minutes, he did not have any GI distress throughout the entire race and felt nutritionally sound from start to finish for the first time in his Ironman racing career.

After the Ironman, our plan called for Mark to drink 20 ounces of sports drink for every pound that he lost during the race (he lost only 2 pounds). We experimented with his recovery drink and nutrient composition throughout his training and concluded that Mark did best if he drank 24 ounces of a recovery drink that had 540 calories, 106 grams of carbohydrates, 26 grams of protein, 2 grams of fat, and various vitamins and minerals.

Mark was then instructed to have a normal mixed meal of carbohydrates, protein, and fat about 2 hours after he drank his recovery drink—his choice was pizza. We did not set any specific amounts of carbohydrates, protein, or fat for this post-race meal because it was time for him to focus on eating for pleasure instead of performance.

Transition Mesocycle (aka Active Recovery)

You've made it through a successful race season and now you are ready to enjoy some much-needed rest and relaxation. Before you do, though, you should note some key nutrition guidelines for this cycle.

Your training intensity obviously has taken a nosedive, as has your training volume. During this cycle you have two goals: (1) rest and recovery and (2) improving sport-specific weaknesses. First things first, though: enjoy some time off (but stay active).

The biggest mistake I see endurance athletes make in this cycle is that they do not decrease the amount of food that they eat. You are used to eating a good amount of food since you are just coming off of your race season and it is often difficult to change the habit of eating every 2–3 hours throughout the day. However, this cycle is infamous for adding unnecessary pounds to an athlete's body. You will most likely gain weight now unless you pay attention to your nutrition and, more importantly, the quantity that you eat. You can easily prevent unwanted weight gain by adopting the following guidelines in addition to decreasing portion sizes and the number of times that you eat during the day.

Daily Macronutrient and Fluid Needs in the Transition Cycle

- **Carbohydrate intake should range from 5–6 g/kg.**

  Nutrition Nibble: Back off on the carbohydrates now and focus more on the color of what you're eating, that is, include more fruits and vegetables with a good amount of fiber.

- **Protein should range from 1.2–1.4 g/kg.**

  Nutrition Nibble: Get back on the program of eating lean meats if you have been supplementing with protein powders and bars through your race season. No need to go crazy with your protein intake since you have virtually no intensity in your training. Just eat enough to promote good health.

- **Fat should range from 0.8–1.0 g/kg.**

  Nutrition Nibble: Be sure to add more sources of essential fatty acids to your eating plan such as oily fish (salmon and mackerel) and flax products.

- **Fluid guidelines are as described in the preparation period.**

  Nutrition Nibble: Hydration is important year-round so don't skimp on your fluid intake. Keep an eye on the color of your urine and use that as your hydration marker.

Table 3.7 has a summary of your daily nutrition needs during this cycle.

Macronutrient and Fluid Timing for Training during the Transition Cycle

You shouldn't be following a formal, structured training program during this cycle but you should be working on any

Table 3.7
Daily Nutrition Needs during the Transition Mesocycle

Training Cycle	Carbohydrate	Protein	Fat	Fluids
Transition	5–6 g/kg	1.2–1.4 g/kg	0.8–1.0 g/kg	enough to produce straw-colored urine

weaknesses that you have, so you will still be training at least a few times per week. You will not need to follow specific timing of nutrient consumption as I recommended for the previous cycles, but it is still extremely important to keep your body well hydrated. Therefore, the following hydration strategies should be followed during this cycle.

- Drink 7–10 ounces of fluid (preferably sports drink) 10–20 minutes before training.
- Drink 7–10 ounces of fluid every 15–20 minutes during training.

  Nutrition Nibble: Since you are watching the amount of calories you eat during this cycle, don't overdo it on the sports drinks. Drinking them is beneficial but just don't go crazy and drink them throughout the day and during your workouts.

- After training, drink 20–24 ounces of fluid for every pound of body weight lost.

  Nutrition Nibble: This principle is still extremely important since dehydration can cause health, as well as performance, problems. Be sure to re-hydrate your body after any training session.

Table 3.8 is a summary of your training needs during this cycle.

Table 3.8
Training Needs during the Transition Mesocycle

Nutrient	Pre-training	During training	Post-training
Fluid	7–10 ounces at 10–20 minutes	7–10 oz. every 15–20 minutes, include sodium	20–24 oz. for every pound of weight lost, include sodium
Carbohydrate	X	X	X
Protein	X	X	X
Fat	X	X	X

General and Specific Eating Guidelines for the Transition Cycle

- **Re-introduce whole foods from all of the food groups.**

  Nutrition Nibble: Chances are you are like most endurance athletes and do not follow an eating program of great variety during your race season. Therefore, it is very important to get back into your "normal" eating habits again and start eating the foods that you haven't been able to in the last few months. Be sure to choose whole foods such as fruits and vegetables to maximize the amount of vitamins and minerals you get and decrease the amount of processed foods.

- **Minimize the use of energy bars, gels, and sports drinks.**

  Nutrition Nibble: Most endurance athletes eat or drink some type of nutrition supplement such as sports drinks, gels, or energy bars 9–10 months out of the year. While there is nothing wrong with that, it does limit the variety of foods you eat and some of these products are high in calories. Put these products in the back of your pantry until your base training cycle begins again.

- **Try new foods and restaurants.**

  Nutrition Nibble: Food should be fun and enjoyable. Too often, athletes get in a rut eating the same foods day in and day out. Be adventurous and try something new. Try new ethnic foods or different preparations of foods you already eat. When you go to a restaurant, don't order what looks familiar or what you usually order. Explore a little and reap the benefits of appreciating different cuisine and nutrients.

- **Don't overeat.**

  Nutrition Nibble: This is by far the most important message to take away during this cycle. You are not training that much, therefore, you are not burning as many calories. You MUST decrease the amount of calories you eat or you will gain unwanted weight. It usually takes about 20 minutes for your brain to get the signal that your stomach is hungry or full. Eat slowly, enjoy your food, don't eat in front of the television, and STOP well before you think you are full. Remember, fluids such as juice, soda, and alcohol have many empty calories that you do not need now, so minimize their consumption.

- **Don't forget about the environment.**

  Nutrition Nibble: If your transition cycle falls in the winter where there is not much sunshine, it is common to eat more comfort foods, which can be very high in calories and tend to increase body weight and body fat. Being aware of this before it happens is the key to avoiding weight gain. Prepare for this by having low-calorie, easy-to-make foods on hand at all times (fruits and vegetables work very well).

SUMMARY

Nutrition periodization is about having a nutrition plan year-round to support your health and training and improve performance. You follow a structured physical training program for at least 9–11 months out of the year and the only way you will be able to make it through your long and high-intensity training days and remain illness-free is to have a well-planned nutrition program that meets your changing needs during each of your periodization cycles.

Don't underestimate the power of nutrition. You are an expert on how your body works and functions so become more in tune with your specific nutrition needs and use the information I presented here to develop your individualized eating program tailored to your health and training.

4

Successful Weight Management

Most endurance athletes would benefit from having a lower body weight for racing, within reason. This is because performance is often negatively impacted when you are carrying a larger mass. It is basic physics and common sense when you think about it. It takes more work and effort to move more mass! However, I would caution you that if you think you should lose weight to improve performance and you are trying to get below a healthy weight for your body, it might negatively impact your performance and health. If you fall into this category, consult a registered dietitian who specializes in sports nutrition first. You cannot race well if you are not healthy. Being at an unhealthy weight will not improve your performance.

Whether it is a good idea for you to lose weight or improve your body composition or not is not the focus of this chapter. That is a question only you can answer for yourself. If you are reading this chapter, I am going to assume that you want to change your body weight and composition in some way and I am going to show you when and how to do it most successfully so that you do not risk illness or sacrifice performance. In terms of how you go about it, it really doesn't make a difference if you want to lose weight for health or performance reasons.

MAKING A LIFESTYLE CHANGE

Let's start by covering the basics of weight or body fat loss. There is no magic pill or crazy fad diet that will speed this process in a safe manner. Sure you can lose 20 pounds in one month, but you will probably put it right back on and them some. Most diets or supplements may help you lose weight and body fat quickly, but the weight loss cannot be maintained because it does not result from a lifestyle change. In order to get to a weight or body composition that you can sustain long-term, you must change the way you approach food and exercise. It doesn't begin with what you eat but with how you think about eating.

The psychology of eating is powerful and I do not intend to provide much information regarding this since I am not a qualified psychologist, but just remember that changing the way your body looks begins in your mind. First you must make the decision to change, then you must implement the changes. If you aren't ready to change your eating style, then you will not be ready to lose weight and body fat and keep it off. When you are ready and motivated and want to change, then you will. Until then, try to make progress toward being ready for change. Start with little changes in your eating program that will improve your overall health, such as increasing the amount of fruits and vegetables that you eat, switching to whole grains, cutting out sodas, or limiting unhealthy fats.

TIMING OF WEIGHT LOSS

Before I describe how to lose weight, it is important for you to know that losing weight during certain times of your training year is not recommended. Restricting the amount of food you eat, resulting in a state of negative energy balance (calories in less than calories out), will impair your performance. This is because eating too few calories could reduce your internal energy stores so that it is harder for you to work out. This could also impair your immune system since you won't be eating as much food with vitamins and minerals. In addition, not eating enough could change your mood so that you do not feel like training. Not training is obviously counterproductive to your goal of losing weight and body fat.

Because of the negative performance impact weight reduction may have, you should only try to actively lose weight during these two cycles of your training year:

- Transition cycle
- The initial part of the preparation cycle

What I mean by actively losing weight is that weight loss is one of your primary goals. You will unintentionally lose and gain a few pounds throughout your training year. Active weight reduction should not be pursued during the end of your preparation cycle because you do not want to enter your speed/strength training with low energy stores, or during your competition cycle because you do not want to undereat when you will be burning many more calories with the speed and interval work that you will perform.

A goal of losing 0.5–1.0 pounds per week is recommended for most endurance athletes to minimize losses of muscle glycogen and lean muscle mass, compromised cardiac function, altered ability to maintain body temperature, and muscle cramping due to electrolyte imbalances. However, during your transition cycle or off-season, you can safely try to lose 1.0–2.0 pounds per week.

Because large changes in scale weight typically reflect changes in fluid balance or glycogen stores, you should focus more on changes in your body composition rather than your total body weight.

One pound of weight or fat loss is equal to 3,500 calories. Therefore, to lose 0.5–1.0 pounds per week, a daily negative energy balance of 250–500 calories must be achieved. Since you will be actively trying to lose weight during your lower volume and intensity training cycles, you should primarily decrease the amount of total food calories to create this calorie deficit. Do this rather than depending on creating a negative calorie balance by expending more energy during training-because it is not going to happen during these training cycles. In addition, non-purposeful general daily activity (non-training) is very important for weight loss. Try to increase the amount of calories you burn in your lifestyle and occupation. I will talk more about this in the next section.

Here are some guidelines regarding how much weight is safe to lose and when it is safe to lose it:

- o Lose 0.5 pounds per week
  - o Recommended in the following cycles:
    - Transition cycle
    - Initial part of preparation cycle
  - o Create a deficit of 250 calories per day

    250 calories per day × 7 days in a week =
    1,750-calorie deficit or 0.5 pounds of weight loss

- o Lose 1.0 pounds per week
  - o Recommended in the following cycles:
    - Transition cycle
    - Initial part of preparation cycle
  - o Create a deficit of 500 calories per day

    500 calories per day × 7 days in a week =
    3,500-calorie deficit or 1.0 pounds of weight loss

- o Lose 1.5 pounds per week
  - o Recommended in the following cycle:
    - Transition cycle
  - o Create a deficit of 750 calories per day

    750 calories per day × 7 days in a week =
    4,250 calorie deficit or 1.5 pounds of weight loss

- o Lose 2.0 pounds per week

    ○ Recommended in the following cycle:
- Transition cycle

    ○ Create a deficit of 1,000 calories per day

$$1{,}000 \text{ calories per day} \times 7 \text{ days in a week} =$$
$$7{,}000\text{-calorie deficit or } 2.0 \text{ pounds of weight loss}$$

BASICS OF WEIGHT LOSS

Overall, losing weight and body fat is really not that difficult when you see it described on paper. The key is to manipulate what I call your Personal Energy Balance Equation (PEBE) so that you are burning more calories than you are eating.

More specifically, if you want to lose weight, you must be in negative energy balance (calories in are less than calories out). So, why is it hard to lose weight and body fat in real life if it looks so easy on paper? The reason is because there are eight different pieces of your PEBE that you must manage. Let's look at this in more detail.

The energy balance equation has two sides: calories in (consumption) and calories out (expenditure), as shown in Figure 4.1. The calories-in side is made up of:

- Carbohydrates
- Protein
- Fat
- Alcohol

This side of the equation is very simple to understand because it is only affected by the amount of food you eat or beverages you drink. The reason that all the food is not lumped together but is separated into four different categories is because each nutrient contributes a different amount of energy per gram.

- Carbohydrates have 4 calories per gram
- Protein has 4 calories per gram

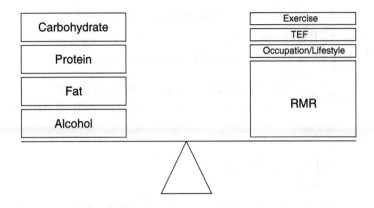

Figure 4.1 The Energy Balance Equation

- Fat has 9 calories per gram
- Alcohol has 7 calories per gram

It is important to take into consideration these differences so that you can choose foods that are lower in total calories when you are trying to lose weight and body fat.

The calories-out side of the equation is much more complicated because biology has more of an impact on each component. These additional factors make it more difficult to balance and manage. It is made up of the following:

- Thermic effect of food (TEF)
- Occupational and lifestyle expenditure
- Exercise expenditure
- Resting metabolic rate

Similar to the calories-in side, each of the four components on the calories-out side has a different contribution to the total amount of calories that you burn or expend.

1. TEF is approximately 10% of your total calories-out. TEF refers to the energy you burn when you consume food and can vary greatly depending on both the quantity and type of food that you eat. TEF is usually not a primary factor in

changing body weight because it doesn't contribute that much to the total calories that you burn. You should just be aware that this happens when you eat and not interpret it as an indication that you should eat more to burn more calories. That simply is not the case and you don't really need to do anything with your TEF. TEF has its own subsets:

- Obligatory thermogenesis, which more simply put is the amount of calories your body burns as it digests and absorbs the food you eat.
- Facultative thermogenesis, which occurs when your nervous system gets activated from eating and increases your metabolism.

2. Occupational/lifestyle expenditure can make up about 10–15% of the total calories that you burn each day. You can have a significant impact on the amount of weight or body fat that you lose by taking advantage of this. What I mean is that no matter what type of job you have or what you do during the day, you have the ability to take more steps, park farther away from the front door, make more trips to the water fountain, and take the stairs. You can do all this without having to plan like you do with your training. The calories you can burn in your normal day outside of training can almost be referred to as "free calories" because you don't have to change clothes or sweat to burn them. The more calories you burn in your daily non-training activities, the more weight or body fat you will lose. The easiest way to increase this type of activity is to use a pedometer or step counter and accumulate a certain amount of steps daily. I will discuss this in more detail later in the chapter.

3. Exercise expenditure is the most variable component of the calories-out side that you have control over. What I mean is that you can burn as few as 5% or as many as 40% of your total calories through exercise depending on what type,

amount, and intensity of training you are doing. Usually it is easier for you to burn these calories because all you have to do is follow your training program.

4. Last but certainly not least is your resting metabolic rate (RMR). RMR is the amount of calories your body burns at rest to perform basic functions such as your heart beating and your brain functioning. This makes up approximately 60–75% of the amount of calories you burn each day. RMR is the most important component on the calories-out side of the energy balance equation because it represents up to three-quarters of the total calories burned by the body. There is good news and bad news about RMR. The good news is that if you know your RMR from having it measured (not predicted from an equation), then you can build an exact calorie budget that will provide you enough energy to train and lose weight and body fat safely. The bad news is that not many athletes know their RMR. As you may know from personal experience, it is very difficult to lose weight. The reason is not necessarily that you have a problem with the amount of calories you eat or burn through your occupation and lifestyle or through your exercise. It may just be that you are trying to lose weight without first knowing how many calories your body needs to survive. Therefore, the amount of calories you eat is a complete guess.

I hope you see why weight loss is a very simple concept on paper but very difficult to actually accomplish. Because you have to balance eight pieces of your PEBE, weight and body fat loss may seem to be an unattainable goal. Actually, you really only have to worry about seven since TEF will not be applicable. I know you may be feeling overwhelmed with this but the reason I presented the different components of your PEBE is for you to have the basic knowledge of what it is going to take to lose the weight or body fat. I am going to show you in this chapter just how easy it is to apply all seven of the components of PEBE that you need to balance, so don't feel overwhelmed with this first round of information.

Before we get into the steps to take to lose weight or body fat, I want to first discuss the weight rebound effect and fad diets.

WHY FAD DIETS DON'T WORK

Now that you have a good understanding of what the energy balance equation is and its different components, let's talk about why fad diets don't work and why 95% of people who go on diets regain the weight they lost and more within 1–2 years. The reason is simple. When you try to lose weight, you either change the composition of your eating, the amount that you eat, the timing of your eating, or the type and amount of exercise that you do. I mentioned it before, but the first step in changing your body is deciding that you are ready to lose the weight or body fat. If you are not ready, you will not succeed.

Once you are ready, it really won't matter how much you change your eating or exercise if you do not know the 60–75% of the calories-out side of the equation that is your resting metabolic rate (RMR). Remember, RMR is the amount of calories that your body needs in a 24-hour period just to survive without food or exercise—even "non-exercise" work like walking from your car to your house. Aside from fad diets being very restrictive in calories and nutrients, one reason that they do not work is because they do not use your measured RMR to determine how many calories you should eat. Estimating your RMR is useless since it is affected by so many different factors that equations don't account for. Specifically, RMR is influenced by:

- Mass—the more you weigh, the higher your RMR. An easy way to think about this is using the analogy of a big SUV versus a smaller, more economical car. The SUV requires and takes more gas to move versus the smaller car. It is the same thing with our body. When we weigh more, we need more calories to survive. When we weigh less, we don't need as many calories to live.

- Body composition—the more muscle you have, the higher your RMR. Muscle burns 2–4 times as many calories as fat does when you are at rest, so the more muscle you have, the more energy you use, even at rest.
- Gender—males usually have higher RMRs because they have more lean muscle mass.
- Genetics—it is believed that RMR can be affected by as much as 30% depending on your genetics.
- Medications—some drugs will increase RMR and others will decrease it.
- Hormones—stress hormones in particular will typically increase your RMR.

As I just mentioned, estimating your RMR based on equations could be very inaccurate and counterproductive to meeting your weight and body fat loss goals. Research has shown that there is a huge range in people's RMR—even people who are of the same physical size. One study, conducted at the University of Pennsylvania in 1988, predicted and measured the RMR of 80 females of the same height and weight. Given their vital statistics you might assume that their RMRs were fairly close to one another. However what the researchers found was shocking to say the least. There was a variance of approximately 500 calories between the predicted and measured RMRs. Because RMR can represent up to 75%, a 500-calorie inaccuracy automatically sets you up for failure before you even start! Why? Well, eating an additional 500 calories daily adds up to a 52-pound weight gain in 1 year!

If you have been unsuccessful in the past with losing weight or body fat, it's probably not because you weren't trying. Most people, when they are ready, are very focused and even though they do slip every so often, they typically stay on the right path. You were unsuccessful because you had no idea of how many calories you should eat to just maintain basic physiological functions. You didn't know your RMR, therefore, you could not accurately determine how many calories you should eat to lose weight and not affect your performance. What should you do now? Have your RMR measured, of course!

MEASURE YOUR RMR

Since the number one factor that influences your RMR is your body mass, a loss of body weight will cause a decrease in your RMR, and vice versa. When you lose weight, your RMR also decreases. This is the explanation for the infamous "yo-yo" dieting phenomenon that happens with people trying to lose weight: they decrease the amount of calories they eat, they may exercise a little, and voila, they lose weight. But their RMR decreases at the same time because they are now at a lower body weight, which isn't a big deal—except when that person looks in the mirror, likes what they see from the weight they have lost, and decides to celebrate by eating a couple of cookies, or going out for drinks with friends, or missing a few training sessions. This person is now increasing the calories-in side of their PEBE and guess what? Their new, lower RMR has a hard time catching back up to support this new increased calorie level. Since RMR cannot catch up at the same rate the calories are going in or not being burned, the person begins to gain weight again.

Therefore, the key factor that will determine how successful you are in losing weight is your RMR. Have your resting metabolic rate measured frequently so you can accurately determine the correct amount of calories you need to eat and the amount of exercise you need to perform in order to reach your weight goals.

Having your RMR measured on a consistent basis is the most important thing you can do when you are trying to lose weight. I cannot stress enough how important it is to get your new RMR measured whenever you lose a significant amount of weight (defined as 5–10% of total body weight) or when you reach a weight-loss plateau (as defined by 5 or more days without weight loss). Even with a modest loss of 5–10 pounds, your body will require fewer calories, which makes it so crucial to readjust your PEBE so that you continue to lose weight.

Enough talk about why you should have your RMR measured. I think I provided a good explanation and argument of why that is so important. Now the question becomes how to measure it.

How Do You Measure Your RMR?

The only true way to have your RMR measured is to visit a performance laboratory or health professional that has an indirect calorimeter, commonly called a metabolic cart. Some companies have actually designed smaller, more portable versions of this that many more health professionals have. Check your local physician's office, a registered dietitian, or a health club to see if they have the capability of measuring your RMR. You can also check with the following companies that manufacture RMR measuring devices:

- HealtheTech, Inc., www.healthetech.com
- Korr, www.korr.com
- New Leaf, www.newleaffitness.com
- Body Media, www.bodymedia.com

What happens when you have your RMR measured is that a machine measures the volume of oxygen (resting VO_2) that you breathe in and out. Because oxygen is needed to break down food for metabolism, measuring it gives you an accurate representation of what your metabolism is. The test itself is very noninvasive since you just have to breathe. It takes from 5–30 minutes and after it is done, you will know exactly how many calories your body needs in a 24-hour period just to maintain itself at its current weight.

After you know that number, you are ready to build your personal calorie budget for weight loss based on your individual physiology without guesswork.

SAFE STEPS TO WEIGHT LOSS: HOW TO DO IT

There are no secrets to weight loss success. Adapting your PEBE to meet you goals is the only thing you need to do to successfully change the way your body looks. The energy balance equation is based on hard science and is your first step in losing weight. Understand your PEBE and all of its components before you embark on the weight loss journey. Of course, there is one catch: you must take personal ownership and be motivated enough to want to make a lifestyle change, rather than a quick fix. The type of weight loss you will see will not be rapid and will not include voiding your eating program of quality nutrients. You will see gradual progress, from 0.5–2.0 pounds of weight loss per week. The good news is that what you won't see is a 5–10 pound or greater weight regain within the first year.

So, if you are ready to make that change and you have the motivation, support from family and friends, and the willingness to change the way your body looks, here are the six steps that you should follow to be successful:

Step 1: Get your RMR measured.
1. Have your RMR measured so you know what your body needs and where to begin.
2. Have your RMR re-measured if you lose 5–10% of your body weight or if you reach a weight plateau of 5 days or longer. Remember, because the number one factor that affects RMR is body mass, as you become smaller, you will not need as many calories, so you will need to readjust your PEBE.

3. One thing to note is the condition in which you have your RMR measured. It is much more accurate to have your RMR measured first thing in the morning after an overnight fast of at least 12 hours. Be sure not to exercise, drink coffee, or eat anything the morning of your test. Prepare for your RMR test just as you would if you were going to have your cholesterol checked.

   a. No matter what the person says who will be measuring your RMR, do not let them measure it if you have not fasted for 12 hours. This is a requirement and if it is not adhered to, it can mean an error of about 100 calories in your RMR.

   b. If you are sick or feeling like you are getting sick, do not have your RMR measured. Illness can cause an elevated RMR measurement.

Step 2: Meet with a registered dietitian (RD).

1. Because you have to try to figure out how all of the components of your PEBE determine your calorie budget, it is best to meet with an RD who specializes in sports nutrition so he or she can help you figure out how many calories you should eat and burn based on your RMR. In addition, the RD can help you determine the correct ratio of carbohydrates, protein, and fat that will help you lose weight and meet your health and performance goals.

2. This person would ideally be the one who will be measuring your RMR, but doesn't have to be.

3. Visit this RD during times of RMR re-measurement and readjustment of your PEBE so he or she can help you modify your calories-in and calories-out based on your new body weight and RMR.

Step 3: Log your foods and beverages.

1. It has been proven that if you write down what you eat, you will be more successful at changing your body weight.

The concept seems to hold people more accountable for their actions and sometimes prevents overeating. Unless you are concerned with other nutrients such as fat, sodium, and cholesterol, you only need to track calories for weight loss.

2. By no means am I proposing that you do this every day of the year. I recommend doing it at first for 1–2 weeks so you begin to learn the amount of calories that are in your normal foods and meals. Once you have a good idea of what each meal or snack provides, you can be fairly accurate in knowing how much you can eat each day without keeping a log.

3. Revisit keeping a food log when you feel that you are losing control. It only takes a quick refresher before you are back on track again.

4. Food logs are extremely beneficial if you will be seeing an RD throughout your weight loss journey. He or she will be able to get a far more accurate representation of how much you are eating if you have an accurate food log.

5. Various software programs exist that can help you accomplish this more easily than the old "pen and paper" method. The benefit of software programs is that you will be able to see your daily progress in real time. You can also use the software program's food database to find calorie counts for common foods and not have to spend the time to search for this information in a calorie reference book. Book or computer, choose whichever fits your lifestyle better. The important thing is that you do it regardless of what method you use.

Step 4: Log your physical activity and exercise and buy a step counter.

1. The same principle applies to entering exercise information into a log as it does to food and beverage. You will be

more successful if you keep track of your exercise to help you know how many calories you are burning.

2. The easiest way to keep track of how many calories you are burning in your occupational and lifestyle activity is to wear a step counter (pedometer).

3. If you walk a total of 10,000 steps per day, you will burn an extra 500 calories per day, without trying that hard. Approximately 2,000 steps are equal to 1 mile of walking and you burn approximately 100 calories per 1 mile walked.

4. If you can achieve a 500-calorie daily deficit in your normal day's activities, then you can lose 1 pound per week without factoring in your nutrition or planned exercise. This is the "free calorie" concept I described earlier. The more you can increase your non-purposeful, occupational or lifestyle activity the more successful you will be at losing weight or body fat.

Step 5: Readjust your PEBE each time you get your RMR re-measured and it is different from the previous time.

1. A significant change in RMR from one measurement to the next is 100–200 calories as long as you have it measured by the same device, the same person, at the same time of day, and under the same fasting conditions. Readjust your PEBE only if your RMR is different by at least 100 calories or more or if you have been at a weight plateau for at least 5 days.

2. If your PEBE is not readjusted with each RMR measurement, it will be impossible for you to remain successful at attaining your weight related goals. For example, one 12-week weight loss study showed that at week 4, participants had lost 8 pounds and RMR had decreased by 89 calories. If the participants did not readjust the amount of calories they ate and expended, they would not continue to lose weight. In fact, the researchers in this study did readjust the energy balance equation at

certain intervals, and at week 12 the average weight loss was 18 pounds with a decrease in RMR of 125 calories. This shows that a very small decrease in RMR can make a big difference in adjusting your PEBE for continuing to lose weight.

Step 6: If you find that you cannot do this on your own, join a program.

1. You just may need a little more help in attaining your goals. Oftentimes, a group setting may help motivate you and keep you on track. Please note that if a group setting intimidates you, do not force yourself into it. You must realize what situation works best for you. If you force yourself into a situation that is not comfortable, you will set yourself up for failure.

2. If a group setting is right for you be sure to look for a program that will provide you the following:

   a. Initial assessment to determine if you are ready to change and take personal ownership of your health by identifying small, incremental steps that will lead you to attaining your long-term goal.

   b. A support network that can be used on a daily basis to help you be successful.

   c. Help with identification of barriers and bypasses.

   d. Participation in group discussion sessions.

3. If a group setting is not your thing, choose a registered dietitian who offers individual consultations. Sometimes it is as easy as meeting with this nutrition professional a few times to get you back on track.

Case Study for Weight Loss

Let's look at an example so you have an idea of how it all fits together.

Cami is a triathlete who focuses on Olympic distance triathlons. She is 5'4" and 150 pounds. She wants to lose 20 pounds at a rate of 1 pound per week; she has just started her 16-week preparation (base training) cycle.

Step 1.

Cami visited a registered dietitian (RD) and had her RMR measured. Her RMR was 1,300 calories per day.

Step 2.

Cami then met with the RD to fill in the remaining components of her PEBE, working on the calories-out side first.

Occupational and lifestyle expenditure: Cami works in an office where she mostly works on a computer, 8 hours per day, 5 days per week so it was determined that the amount of calories that she burned during work were minimal. For a relatively sedentary occupation, the amount of calories burned will be around 600.

Exercise expenditure: Cami trains 6 days per week. She swims 3 hours per week, bikes 3 hours per week, runs 3 hours per week and strength trains for 2 hours per week. Based on these amounts of planned exercise, Cami will burn approximately:

- Swim: 1,450 calories per week
- Bike: 2,500 calories per week
- Run: 2,600 calories per week
- Strength training: 450 calories per week

Cami's total calories burned through exercise are 7,000 each week or 1,000 calories per day. There are many books and Web sites that provide you with the tools to calculate how many calories you will burn when you exercise.

Thermic effect of food: Remember that we will not figure TEF into the equation.

Resting metabolic rate: Cami's RMR was measured in Step 1 at 1,300 calories per day.

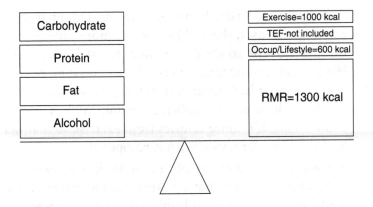

Figure 4.2 Cami's PEBE

After determining that Cami burns 2,900 calories per day (1,300 from her RMR, 600 from her occupation, 1,000 from her exercise), it was time to determine how many calories she should eat per day.

To lose 1 pound per week, Cami must accumulate a deficit of 3,500 calories each week, which is a deficit of 500 calories per day. Cami and the RD determined that she is currently burning 2,900 calories per day so by decreasing the amount of calories she eats to 2,400, Cami will be in a negative energy balance or deficit of 500 calories per day.

Cami's Plan

Calories-in: 2,400   Calories-out: 2,900

A 500-calorie daily deficit will equal 1 pound of weight loss per week. Some things to keep in mind about this example:

1. Because Cami is beginning her preparation cycle, which will include lower volume and intensity, she will not need to eat as many calories. Once her training volume begins to increase throughout this cycle, she can begin to even out the deficit between the calories that she eats and the calories

that she burns. Basically, as her duration and intensity of training increases, she will be burning more calories through exercise so she doesn't have to eat 500 calories less per day. As she trains more, she will need more calories to support her training, therefore, she should create her 500-calorie per day deficit by eating 250 less calories and burning 250 more calories from exercise so that her health and performance are not hampered.

2. In this example, Cami's specific macronutrient composition (calories from carbohydrate, protein, and fat) was not configured. This is because this is highly individual and based on many different factors that must be discussed with a registered dietitian.

Step 3.

Now that Cami knows exactly how many calories she should eat based on her individual RMR, she can begin to apply this information as she makes food choices. Cami has a couple of options:

• The first is to purchase a software food-logging program where she can log all of her food and beverage intake using a computer. This is a nice option because it provides much more accurate data, however, it is not a good fit for some athletes. Determine if using a computer fits your lifestyle and personality.

• What I usually recommend is that the athlete read nutrition labels found on the foods they eat and write down the calorie content per serving that they eat for about 5–7 days (refer to the sample food diary in the appendix). This exercise will teach the athlete the calorie content of common foods and will allow them to keep track of their calorie levels. I also recommend doing this exercise every 2–4 weeks as a refresher and to make sure that the athlete still has a good grasp of the calories that they are eating.

Step 4.

Cami can log her exercise via a computer software program or she can use the pencil-and-paper method.

- If using the pencil-and-paper method, the numbers will not be as accurate, so I recommend at least using an online resource that provides calories burned for different exercises.

Cami can easily keep track of her occupational activity calories burned by wearing a step counter. A step counter worn throughout the day will provide her the amount of calories that her body burns doing what is called non-purposeful activity (basically, anything but exercise). In general, 2,000 steps are equal to one mile of walking and 100 calories are burned for each mile walked.

- Looking at this in more detail, if Cami were to log 10,000 steps each day, she would burn an additional 500 calories from her daily activity, which would provide her 1 pound of weight loss per week without changing the amount of food that she eats.
- Paying attention to daily steps is the easiest way to lose weight because you do not have to decrease the amount of food you eat or increase the amount of exercise you do. By simply getting 10,000 steps per day, you could lose 1 pound per week.

Step 5.

Eight weeks have passed and Cami has lost 10 pounds. She has her RMR measured again to discover that it is 1,200 calories. This is completely normal, remember, since the number one predictor of RMR is body mass.

With her new RMR, she visits the RD again to readjust her PEBE so that she does not get stuck on a weight plateau and so that she does not start gaining weight.

With her new RMR of 1,200 calories, if Cami were to eat the same amount of calories and not increase her exercise, she would be in a positive energy balance of 100 calories per day. This would cause her to regain the weight because she did not readjust her PEBE with her new RMR.

Step 6.

This step (join a program or seek individual weight coaching) would need to be taken only if Cami was not seeing success in the first 3–4 weeks.

Cami noted that she did not like group settings so she would look to the RD who helped her throughout the initial steps to help her stay on track with individual consultations.

SUMMARY

There you have it: six concrete guidelines to follow for weight loss. Unless you have a chronic disease or medical condition, you should not void your eating program of certain foods. That is just not necessary. Your goal should be to enjoy food and control your weight and PEBE based on your individual metabolism, not to restrict yourself to eating only certain foods. Eating healthy should be fun, not a chore. Develop good lifestyle habits and reap the rewards of a new body!

5

Nutrition Supplementation

Should I take it? Do I need it? Is it healthy? Is it safe? Does it work? How much does it cost?

These are the most common questions I hear from athletes about nutritional supplements. I will address most of these questions in this chapter and help you determine if you should add a nutritional supplement to your daily eating program. The nutritional supplements I am referring to include sports drinks, recovery products, energy bars, energy gels, and various vitamin and mineral supplements. What is not included in this chapter are ephedra, steroids, or supplements that are aimed more toward the strength or power athlete because most endurance athletes do not bother with those as they do not improve endurance.

This chapter is not meant to contain the same material as you find in the rest of the sports nutrition books in the bookstores. I will not be covering specific supplements and whether or not you should use them. Rather, I will provide you with often-overlooked information about some of the key ingredients that manufacturers use in sports drinks, energy bars, energy gels, and recovery drinks. If you have an understanding of what types of ingredients are used in your favorite products and in products that you are thinking of trying, you will have a better understanding about how they work in your body and you can decide which ones are right for you and your specific needs. But, first, let's take a look at nutritional supplements in general.

THE NUTRITION SUPPLEMENTS MARKET

Nutrition supplements are very popular among endurance athletes, to say the least. As many as 75% of athletes take some type of supplement—ranging from a simple multivitamin to a complex assortment of pills and powders. The nutritional supplement category is large but I am going to focus on those that are specifically marketed to you, the endurance athlete. In the first part of this chapter, I will discuss a quite alarming topic of supplement contamination that is very prominent these days. I will then move on to how to choose a supplement, nutrition quackery, and finally a discussion of which supplements may offer you an ergogenic (performance-enhancing) effect.

Open up an endurance athlete's pantry and I can almost guarantee that you will find a bottle of multivitamins, a tub of a sports drink or recovery beverage, a few boxes of energy bars or gels, and possibly even some "mystery" supplements that claim to improve performance but really don't.

Supplement Basics

The Dietary Supplements Health and Education Act (DSHEA) of 1994 stated that nutritional supplements that do not claim to diagnose, prevent, or cure disease are not subject to regulation by the Food and Drug Administration (FDA). Unfortunately many supplement manufacturers have concluded that DSHEA guidelines mean that there is no need for them to prove claimed benefits, to show safety with acute or chronic administration, to commit to accepted quality assurance practices, or to follow the stringent labeling regulations followed for food products.

The nutritional supplement industry represents a $2 billion a year growth industry with total global revenue sales projected to be in excess of $4.5 billion by 2007. Athletes from around the world are turning to nutritional supplements as a way to get bigger, faster, and stronger and to get any possible edge over their competition. However, what athletes do not know—or are finding out the hard way—is that many of the supplements on the shelves do not contain the advertised amounts of substances in them, or, even worse, have additional substances in them that are not listed on the label. This can be of particular concern if you have health issues where a certain herb or manufactured supplement could interfere with medications that you may be taking.

Supplement Contamination

Quality assurance for dietary supplements continues to be a concern. Some companies follow good manufacturing practices (GMPs), but others do not. It is hard for athletes to know what products contain, especially when you consider that contamination of a supplement can occur at so many levels in the supply and manufacturing process. Avoiding all products of companies that produce and sell prohormones such as nandrolone and testosterone derivatives, which result in positive drug tests, may not be enough to prevent purchase of contaminated products.

Since the release of the Schanzer report commissioned by the International Olympic Committee in 1999, which stated that 18% of all dietary supplements may lead to a positive doping offence, there has been increasing commercial awareness of the adverse publicity companies face if they are connected with contaminated products. As you will see later in this section, these products are not limited to supplements that strength/power athletes would be taking. You may be surprised to see some of the common supplements you take may be at risk for supplement contamination.

The problem is clearly widespread, as indicated by an investigation conducted by the International Olympic Committee laboratory in Cologne, Germany. During 2000 and 2001, 634 supplements were purchased from 13 different countries and tested. Of these, 94 supplements (14.8% of the total) contained prohibited substances. It was indicated that in another 10% steroids may have been present but the analysis was not conclusive. These results point to a one in four risk of contamination with prohibited substances!

Products that tested positive were purchased in the Netherlands (26%), Austria (23%), the United States (19%), the United Kingdom (19%), Italy (14%), Spain (14%), and Germany (12%), among others. Contamination levels of products tended to be small and highly variable among and within batches, making it difficult to identify the source of the contaminated supplement. Even though the prohibited substances that were found have not been officially published, they included the following types and/or categories:

- Branched-chain amino acids (popular among endurance athletes)
- Glutamine (popular among endurance athletes)
- Zinc (popular among endurance athletes)
- Chrysin
- Tribulus terrestris
- Vitamins (popular among endurance athletes)
- Minerals (popular among endurance athletes)
- Creatine
- Ribose
- Conjugated linoleic acid
- Carnitine
- Guarana

- Pyruvate
- Beta-hydroxy-beta-methylbutyrate (HMB)
- Protein powders (popular among endurance athletes)
- Herbal extracts

There are several industry-driven GMP programs in place, though many experts continue to be concerned about sources of raw materials and guarantees for each batch of product. One industry program is overseen by the National Nutritional Foods Association (NNFA), which has certified dozens of companies and has a strategic alliance with NSF International (www.nsf.org). Membership in NNFA requires compliance with its GMPs, and its Web site (www.nnfa.org) lists companies that are members. NSF International has an athlete-certification program, and can test specific products for interested athletes. Two other resources include ConsumerLabs.com, which has independently tested dietary supplements and has an Athletic Banned Substances Screened Products Program, and the FDA, which has also presented an outline of a GMP program on its website at www.cfsan.fda.gov.

I am not advocating avoiding all products designed to help the athlete nutritionally. It would be hard to imagine completing a long training session without the replacement of carbohydrate, fluid, and electrolytes, and the products that provide these ingredients are vital to training and competition. However, it is important to exercise caution when choosing supplements as any product can be contaminated and there aren't any industry standards in place to prevent this. The good news is that the industry is moving toward standardization, but it will surely take time.

What to Look for and What to Avoid!

As an endurance athlete, you are faced with many new supplements that claim to improve aerobic capacity, buffer lactic acid, decrease muscle soreness, increase power, improve recovery, improve immune function, etc. This list goes on and on! The sixty-four-thousand-dollar question is, "Which ones really work?" There are a few ergogenic (performance-enhancing) aids that have withstood the rigors of time and scientific testing whose claims have been substantiated, but a majority of ergogenic aids have no proven research to support their claims.

The following is a 12-step checklist to help you decide if a product is truly worth buying. If you answer yes to any of these questions, then you should be skeptical of such supplements and investigate further before investing any money.

1. Does the product promise quick improvement in health or physical performance?
2. Does it contain some secret ingredient or formula?
3. Is it advertised mainly with anecdotes, case histories, or testimonials?
4. Are currently popular personalities or star athletes featured in its advertisements?
5. Does it take a simple truth about a nutrient and exaggerate that truth in terms of health or physical performance?
6. Does it question the integrity of the scientific or medical establishment?
7. Is it advertised in a health or sports magazine whose publishers also sell nutritional aids?
8. Does the person who recommends it also sell the product?
9. Does it use the results of a single study or outdated and poorly-controlled research to support its claims?
10. Is it expensive, especially when compared to the cost of obtaining the equivalent nutrients from ordinary foods?
11. Is it a recent discovery not available from any other source?
12. Are the claims too good to be true or does it promise the impossible?

Take these questions into consideration the next time you are looking for that nutritional edge to enhance your performance or health. Not all ergogenic aids or nutritional supplements are useless but a good majority of them are. There may be some products out there that may help you become a better athlete, but do your research first to make sure the product is safe and that it actually holds true to the claims it is making.

One last thing to note is that supplement companies do not have to prove a supplement's safety, effectiveness, or potency before placing a product on the market. Manufacturers of supplements are not supposed to make unsubstantiated health claims about their products but easily get around this stipulation with the following disclaimer: *This statement has not been evaluated by the Food and Drug Administration. This product is not intended to diagnose, treat, cure, or prevent disease.* If you see these words on a label, investigate further.

So, you have decided that a supplement may be right for you, but how do you choose which one? Although there are no guarantees, you will be safer if you select dietary supplements that meet the following criteria:

- **Carry USP (United States Pharmacopoeia) on the label.** "USP" on the label means that the supplement passes tests for dissolution (how well it dissolves), disintegration, potency, and purity. The manufacturer should also be able to demonstrate that the product passes tests for content potency, purity, and uniformity.
- **Made by nationally known food and drug manufacturers.** Reputable manufacturers follow strict quality control procedures. If the company does not answer questions or address complaints, do not use their product.
- **Supported by research.** Reputable companies should provide research from peer-reviewed journals to support claims.
- **Accurate and appropriate claims.** If statements are unclear or the label makes preposterous claims, it is unlikely the company follows good quality control procedures. If the claims sound too good to be true, be wary.

There you have it. Buyer beware!

NUTRITION SUPPLEMENTS FOR THE ENDURANCE ATHLETE

The following information will provide you with a good understanding of some of the ingredients found in the nutrition supplements that you may be using or plan to use in the future. This will allow you to evaluate each ingredient and decide if it is right for your body and training needs.

Sports Drinks

There are so many sports drinks these days that it is very confusing which one to choose. There are products that have been around for 30 or more years and products that have only been introduced to endurance athletes in the last few years. The biggest variables between all of these sports drinks include:

1. **The type of sugar or sugars used**

   As you will see later in this section, there are many types of sugars that are used in sports drinks. The most common include sucrose, glucose, and fructose. The type of sugar affects sweetness. Sweetness can reduce fluid intake. High fructose levels can cause gastrointestinal distress because they slow absorption. Multiple carbohydrate sources, such as the combination of sucrose and glucose and, to a lesser degree, fructose, help stimulate fluid absorption. Using more than one type of carbohydrate source allows manufacturers to use various textures and taste combinations. It might also benefit digestion to have various types of carbohydrates in a drink, as they all use slightly different transport mechanisms when being absorbed across the small intestine.

2. **The carbohydrate concentration**

   Research has shown that a sports drink with 6–8 % carbohydrate concentration is well absorbed and utilized by the body for energy. In fact, Gatorade, which has a 6% carbohydrate concentration, empties from the stomach just as quickly as water. Anything above 8% will delay emptying from the stomach and could cause stomach problems.

3. The osmolality

Osmolality is a term referring to the number of particles in a solution. A solution with fewer particles (low osmolality) tends to produce faster fluid absorption. High osmolality (>400) can slow fluid absorption. As an example, Gatorade has an osmolality range of 280–360 and is emptied from the stomach just as quickly as water.

4. The sodium content

A sodium level of about 110 milligrams per 8 ounces enhances taste, optimizes absorption, and maintains body fluids. Generally speaking, the lower sodium levels in water and some sports drinks may not stimulate voluntary drinking or help maintain fluid balance as does the higher sodium content in other sports drinks. With the increased prevalence of hyponatremia among endurance athletes, I would recommend choosing a sports drink with at least 200 milligrams of sodium per 8 ounces.

If you are wondering about vitamins and minerals added to sports drinks, don't spend too much time analyzing it. No data exist to show physiological benefits of adding any vitamins to a sports drink. In fact, some B vitamins adversely affect the taste of a beverage and could actually decrease the amount you drink.

Sugar in Sports Drinks

Most of the attention surrounding sports drinks is paid to the type of sugar used. Since most quality sports drinks have the same basic formula of electrolytes plus carbohydrate, to differentiate themselves, manufacturers talk about their special sugar or special combination of sugars. Most sports drinks have a combination of one or more of the following sugars:

- Sucrose
- Fructose
- High fructose corn syrup
- Glucose
- Dextrose
- Galactose
- Maltodextrin
- Glucose polymers

Each one could have the potential to upset your stomach depending on the duration or intensity of your event, the environmental conditions, and your individual likes and dislikes. Let's take a closer look at each.

- Sucrose is a disaccharide (made up of two simple sugars) and is common table sugar. It is made up of one glucose unit and one fructose unit. It is extracted from sugar cane and beet sugar and is the most common disaccharide in the diet.
- Fructose is the simple sugar found in fruit and honey and is sweeter than common table sugar. It is digested more slowly because it must first pass through the liver to be broken down into glucose.
- High fructose corn syrup is an especially sweet corn syrup. It differs from traditional corn syrup in that 45–55% of its carbohydrate is enzymatically hydrolyzed to the simple sugars glucose and fructose. It is less viscous than traditional corn syrup but has nearly twice the concentration of mono- and disaccharides than regular corn syrup. It is the predominant sweetener found in commercially sweetened foods.
- Glucose is the main carbohydrate found in the blood and is used to make the glycogen stored in the liver and muscle. It is the main carbohydrate energy source in the body's cells
- Glucose polymers are long molecular chains with glucose as the fundamental building block. Glucose polymers are glucose

chain sugars that are not as sweet as sucrose or corn syrup that is commonly found in cola-type drinks. These glucose polymers provide a greater amount of energy without being too sweet.

- Dextrose is another name for glucose.
- Galactose is a monosaccharide but does not stimulate an insulin response directly. Similar to fructose, galactose must first visit the liver to be broken down into glucose.
- Maltodextrin is a glucose polymer that is manufactured by breaking long starch units into smaller ones. It is also found frequently in processed foods. It is considered a complex carbohydrate.

There is only one additional topic to discuss when it comes to the types of sugar found in sports drinks. Each sugar has a different glycemic index value, which means that it will be digested faster or slower. Choosing the wrong sports drink based on its sugar has the potential to cause serious stomach problems. Glycemic index of foods can be affected by many different variables such as preparation method, protein and fat presence, fiber content, and more. What I am going to present is the glycemic index information based on single sugars that are found in sports drinks. It is very rare to find a food that has only one sugar in it that won't be affected by the other factors that affect its glycemic index value. I will discuss the glycemic index in much more detail in Chapter 6.

High glycemic index sugars are rapidly absorbed into the blood and provide an immediate source of energy. Low glycemic index sugars are absorbed more slowly and provide a delayed source of muscle energy. Examples of high glycemic index sugars in sports drinks are:

- Sucrose
- Glucose (dextrose)
- Maltodextrin
- Glucose polymers

Examples of low glycemic index sugars are:

- Fructose
- Galactose

Lower glycemic index carbohydrates such as fructose and galactose are well-tolerated when they are in combination with another sugar in a sports drink but not by themselves. When large concentrations of fructose are consumed during exercise, it can result in gastrointestinal discomfort and diarrhea. A small amount of fructose in a sports drink won't cause problems as long as there are other more easily absorbed sugars (i.e., ones that are high glycemic) also present.

You may find other ingredients in some sports drinks, including protein, green tea extract, magnesium, calcium, and vitamins, but the main components that have a large impact on performance have already been discussed. These secondary nutrients are generally not as important in sports drinks since they don't serve a predominant role. However, the addition of protein to sports drinks has become a hot topic so I want to provide you some baseline knowledge about it so you can make an informed choice.

Protein in Sports Drinks

Protein has been very popular among endurance athletes lately and I want to provide you a good understanding of why some manufacturers put it in their products and whether or not it will be useful to you.

It has been suggested that consuming a protein-carbohydrate mixture during exercise will raise blood insulin to higher levels than carbohydrate alone. Having a higher blood insulin level would increase the body's use of carbohydrate in muscle and better delay fatigue. The hormone insulin is responsible for transporting carbohydrate from the blood into the muscle cell where it can be used for energy.

Pro & Carb ⇒ ↑ insulin ⇒ ↑ muscle uptake glucose ⇓ energy / delay fatigue

Research has shown that consuming carbohydrate during exercise delays fatigue by increasing the amount of energy that is supplied by blood glucose, thereby slowing the rate of muscle glycogen depletion. During long exercise sessions of more than 90 minutes, if carbohydrate is in short supply protein can contribute up to 15% of your total energy but if you are replenishing your carbohydrate stores at consistent intervals, protein use is minimal. There have been a few research studies that have shown that the consumption of protein during training can provide additional benefits. These benefits include:

1. A stronger insulin response

Some preliminary research has shown that a small amount of protein added to carbohydrates results in a stronger insulin response, which allows glucose to be delivered to the muscles faster. This, in turn, conserves stored muscle glycogen that can be used at a later time and may delay fatigue.

2. Reduced muscle protein breakdown

As I mentioned earlier, in longer training sessions of 90 minutes or more, protein can be used as an energy source if carbohydrates are not being constantly replenished. The protein that would be used as energy would come from muscle proteins, which means your muscles would be breaking down to a certain extent to provide your body the energy to keep exercising.

While the benefits of protein seem positive, the research to prove this is still in its infancy so I would recommend that if you want to try this protein-carbohydrate mix, do it in your longer training sessions before trying it in a race. Some athletes I have worked with swear by it while others have had serious stomach problems. I will not make a recommendation whether or not you should include it in your training until more research proves the benefits without ill effects in different environments, sports, intensity levels, and athletes.

How to Read a Sports Drink Label

This next section may seem a bit trivial but if you don't know how to properly read a label on a sports drink, you will not be able to determine if the amounts of carbohydrate present are beneficial for you and your training and racing needs. I know label reading seems basic, but this is different than reading a nutrition facts label that you find on other foods. As you will see, there is a bit of mathematics that you must do before you find your answers, so grab a calculator, a piece of paper, and a pencil.

- Look for sports drinks with 14 grams of carbohydrate per 8-ounce serving to encourage rapid fluid replenishment (this is a 6% carbohydrate).
- To calculate the carbohydrate concentration of any beverage as a percentage, divide the amount of carbohydrate (in grams) in one serving by the amount of fluid (in milliliters) in one serving. Then multiply by 100.
  o Example:

$$\frac{14 \text{ grams of carbohydrate} \times 100}{240 \text{ milliliters}} = 5.83 \text{ or } 6\%$$

Choosing the Right Sports Drink for You

Now that you know the different types of sugars found in sports drinks and how to figure out the carbohydrate concentration in these drinks, we can answer the ever-popular question of which one you should choose.

It is a fairly simple question to answer. Aside from having sugars that are easy for you to digest, the right amount of sodium, and the right carbohydrate concentration, the best sports drink is the one that you can tolerate at full concentration (as stated on the mixing instructions) and that you like the most. If you dilute a sports drink in order to tolerate it, you will most likely not get enough carbohydrates and sodium, which is defeating the purpose of using a sports drink. If you don't like the taste, you will not keep drinking it, which results in a greater risk of dehydration and hyponatremia.

Energy Bars

There is quite a variety of energy bars on the market now, ranging from low-calorie and low-carbohydrate bars to meal-replacement bars. There are some significant differences among them besides the obvious variations in calories, carbohydrate, protein, and fat content. You should be aware of these differences before choosing a bar for yourself. However, you would only know this if you read the fine print found in a not-so-convenient location on the wrapper. I am referring to the ingredients list.

How many times do you read the nutrition facts label but not the ingredients list? I am guessing that this happens quite often because we usually don't need too much information from the ingredients list since we can see the breakdown of macro- and micronutrients on the nutrition facts label. However, I urge you to read the ingredients list before making the final decision to choose an energy bar. Why? Because some of the ingredients are actually not healthy! I know it seems odd to find unhealthy ingredients in an energy bar but it is the case with many energy bars.

Here is a list of some of the more popular ingredients found in some energy bars. Remember that ingredients are listed on the label in order of their presence; this means that any ingredient listed in the top three is present in large quantities.

Fractionated Palm Kernel Oil

As you may remember from Chapter 3, palm kernel oil is predominantly a saturated fat and is not healthy. When the palm oil is fractionated, it has a higher concentration of saturated fat than regular palm oil. In this form it is used for the convenience of manufacturers, who like its stability and melting characteristics.

Be aware that fractionated palm kernel oil is in many of the energy bars on the market, usually found in the coating or icing.

From a health perspective, it would be good idea to limit bars containing this in your diet.

Sugar Alcohols

"Zero impact carbs" or "net carbs": more than likely you have heard these terms because they are used very often in our newly carbohydrate-conscious society. What these terms are referring to is the use of sugar alcohols. Sugar alcohols, also known as polyols, are ingredients used as sweeteners and bulking agents. They occur naturally in foods and come from plant products such as fruits and berries. As a sugar substitute, they provide fewer calories (about one-half to one-third less calories) than regular sugar. This is because they are converted to glucose more slowly, require little or no insulin to be metabolized, and don't cause sudden increases in blood sugar.

Sugar alcohols help to provide the sweet flavor in some energy bars. If a manufacturer uses the term "sugar free" or "no added sugar," they must list the grams of sugar alcohols on the label. If more than one sugar alcohol is used in a product, the "Nutrition Facts" panel will list the total amount of sugar alcohol that product contains under the total carbohydrate. Common sugar alcohols are mannitol, sorbitol, xylitol, lactitol, isomalt, maltitol, and hydrogenated starch hydrolysates (HSH).

There are some negatives associated with eating bars containing sugar alcohols. The most common side effects include the possibility of bloating and diarrhea. Both of these are definitely not things that you want to experience during a longer training session or race. If you want to eat bars with sugar alcohols, don't do it during training or a race.

Glycerin (Glycerine, Glycerol)

Glycerin, a commercial product whose principal component is glycerol, is not technically a carbohydrate, though it does contain about the same number of calories per gram. Glycerin is a type of alcohol that is one of the by-products of fat metabolism. The interesting thing about glycerin in some energy bars is that manufacturers include it but do not count its contribution to calorie and carbohydrate totals on the label. What this means is that there may be more carbohydrates and calories than what is stated. One energy bar that the manufacturer stated contained only 2 grams was tested by ConsumerLabs.com and was found to have 20 additional grams of carbohydrate from glycerin. Quite a significant difference! My recommendation for you is buyer beware, since all of the calories may not be reported on the labels of products that contain glycerin.

Caffeine

Caffeine stimulates the central nervous system, which releases adrenaline. Adrenaline increases the use of body fat as a fuel source by mobilizing free fatty acids and thus spares stored carbohydrate so it can be used later in exercise. While caffeine may seem to be a very beneficial ingredient to have in an energy bar, it is classified as a diuretic that may dehydrate you if you are not drinking adequate fluids and can also cause bowel movements and stomach pain. All of the consequences of consuming caffeine far outweigh any benefits. You want to get to the finish line feeling good, not having to deal with digestive problems. In addition, caffeine is a thermogenic compound, which means it increases your heart rate and core body temperature. If you are training or racing in any type of warm environment, this could be detrimental to your performance.

If you are a normal user of caffeine, you will not see any positive impact on performance due to caffeine use because your body builds up a tolerance to caffeine over time. You can cycle caffeine so you do not consume any for 4–5 days before a race then introduce it the day before the competition, but the negative effects (headaches) you get from doing this are probably not worth it.

Green Tea Extract

Green tea is associated with a mild increase in thermogenesis, which means that it increases the amount of calories that you burn. This is due mostly to its caffeine content and it is relatively safe to consume. However, if a bar contains green tea extract and it does in fact increase the amount of calories that you burn, it would not be beneficial to eat during exercise because you already have a hard enough time trying to replenish lost calories. Adding more lost calories that you have to try to replenish somehow is counterproductive during exercise.

Fiber

Fiber content in grams is always reported on the nutrition facts label. As you know, fiber is a very healthy nutrient that is a necessity in your normal eating program. However, when present in larger amounts, it could cause more bathroom breaks than you want to take during training and could be a huge burden during a race. For the days leading up to an important training session or race, try to minimize the use of bars with a larger amount of fiber if you know that higher fiber encourages you to stop often.

Other Things to Consider

It is said that knowledge is power. I believe this statement is true because increasing your knowledge about the less-popular ingredients in energy bars will allow you to have more power in choosing the right energy bar for your body and training.

One last note before we move on: don't forget to look at the very fine print on energy bar labels where it states if the product was manufactured on equipment that processes nuts, wheat, and seeds or if it may contain peanuts or traces of other nuts. If you are allergic to nuts or seeds or are sensitive to gluten (wheat), you will want to avoid bars with these warnings.

Energy Gels

I think of energy gels as a mix between a sports drink and an energy bar. The primary purpose of energy gels is to provide you carbohydrates that can be used for immediate use to fuel your working muscles. Unfortunately, many manufacturers of energy gels believe that more is better and begin adding nutrients that are simply not necessary during exercise. They usually extrapolate from one or two nutrient success stories to believe that the addition of nutrients would benefit the entire gel. Not only does this not produce the effects they hope for but it can also alter taste. As I mentioned in the section about sports drinks, a product must taste good to you in order for you to keep consuming it and reap the benefits of using it.

What I will say about energy gels is to look at the sugar first to see if it is the type that you want for your training or race. There are two sugars that are used in some energy gels that are different from the traditional glucose and maltodextrins: honey and brown rice syrup.

Honey

Honey is primarily a combination of the natural sugars fructose and glucose (38% and 31%, respectively). The third major component of honey is water, accounting for approximately 17%. It is a natural sweetener and is typically easy to digest but takes longer to get into the bloodstream.

Brown Rice Syrup

Brown rice syrup is a polysaccharide (complex carbohydrate) and is digested and released into the bloodstream more slowly than simple sugars. It is a thick amber syrup made by combining sprouted barley with cooked brown rice and fermenting it in a warm environment.

Choosing an Energy Gel

Remember, supplying your body with quick-acting carbohydrates is the primary purpose of energy gels so you don't need to focus much attention on the other additives such as sodium, potassium, amino acids, and green tea extract. You should depend on your sports drink for the first two and don't need to worry too much about the last two unless you want to experiment with added protein to your training or race day nutrition.

Recovery Drinks

Before I discuss recovery drinks, I should say that it is possible to get the same nutrients from food. You just have to know what is required in the recovery nutrition "window of opportunity" and which foods have those nutrients. Having said that, some athletes simply cannot eat food after exercise or have travel schedules that will not allow for easy access to food. This is when the "mix with water" recovery drinks come in very handy.

Only a few really good recovery drinks have entered the market in the past few years, and some of the others should not even be on the market. The drinks that have solid scientific research to support them are the leaders by far but even if they have science on their side, it doesn't guarantee that they will taste good. The real dilemma for you becomes, which recovery drink has what you actually need in it to help your recovery and still tastes good enough to buy? These are two very important questions because some of the ingredients in some of the recovery drinks simply do not need to be in there.

Let's discuss that in a bit more detail. Training and racing introduces a great amount of stress to your body. It depletes your glycogen stores, increases the amount of cortisol in your body (see Chapter 6 for more information about cortisol), and decreases the essential vitamins and minerals in your body.

The Window of Opportunity

Research has shown that there is a 30-minute window immediately following exercise when insulin sensitivity is at its highest and muscles are more apt to accept nutrients. If the nutrients that you eat or drink are not absorbed quickly or are not present in the right amounts during that window, the opportunity for maximum restoration will be lost.

The primary goals for a solid recovery nutrition plan are to replenish the following:

1. Muscle glycogen
2. Body water
3. Electrolytes

The depletion of muscle glycogen can happen quickly during a training session. In fact, it is not uncommon for an athlete weighing 130–160 pounds to lose the following after a hard training session or race:

1. 70 ounces of water (range 35–123 ounces)
2. 5 grams of sodium chloride
3. 200 grams of muscle glycogen
4. 50 grams of liver glycogen

Muscle Glycogen

We have known for years that the restoration of muscle glycogen is an important factor in proper recovery from training. However for a long time the proper mixture of macronutrients was not scrutinized for the basis of recovery nutrition. Recently, the role of protein has taken center stage and there is some fairly decent research to support its role in recovery nutrition.

The hormone insulin regulates glycogen replenishment. Insulin increases the transport of glucose from the blood into the muscle and stimulates the enzyme responsible for the conversion of glucose to glycogen. Insulin is also reported to stimulate the transport of amino acids into the muscle, thereby speeding the protein rebuilding process following exercise. In addition, insulin is reported to blunt the rise in cortisol (the hormone responsible for protein breakdown) following exercise, helping to maintain muscle protein.

Recent research has proven that consuming protein with a carbohydrate source rather than just a carbohydrate alone during recovery is beneficial. In fact, one study showed that the addition of protein to carbohydrate post-training led to a more rapid replenishment of glycogen. Test subjects who consumed protein with carbohydrate measured slightly higher in glycogen restoration at 4 hours post-training than those who consumed carbohydrate alone. Several other research studies found a reduction of total free radical buildup (by 69%), increased insulin levels (by 70%), decreased post-exercise muscle damage (by 36%), and increased muscle glycogen levels (2.2-fold). There is no doubt that the addition of protein to recovery nutrition is important and useful for endurance athletes.

Current recommendations to enhance glycogen re-synthesis post-training include eating 1.0–1.2 grams of rapidly absorbed carbohydrate per kilogram of body weight (i.e., glucose) and 6–20 grams of protein within the first 30 minutes after the completion of exercise. Continue this every 2 hours until the next complete meal. Hydrolyzed whey protein (found in some recovery drinks but not all, so read the ingredients list first) may be one of the best types of protein to eat after exercise because it is predigested and absorbed more quickly. In addition, whey protein isolate used in some recovery drinks is another good choice because it has the highest biological value of proteins and contains branched-chain amino acids, which are important for repairing muscle tissue and for immune system protection.

The amino acid glutamine, which is found in almost every recovery product, is also beneficial to include in your nutrition recovery protein make-up. Intense exercise decreases glutamine stores faster than the body can replenish them. When this happens, the body breaks down muscle tissue. Research has shown that glutamine supports glycogen and protein synthesis and increases nitrogen retention, making it essential for muscle repair.

Body Water and Electrolyte Restoration

Complete re-hydration requires both enough sodium replacement and extra water intake beyond that which is lost in sweat and urine during training. Electrolytes can accelerate re-hydration by speeding the absorption of fluids and improving fluid retention.

It is recommended to consume a sports drink with adequate sodium (at least 110 milligrams per 8 ounces but ideally 200 milligrams per 8 ounces) to match weight loss or drink large volumes of fluid and eat foods that contain a sufficient amount of salt (approximately 3–6 grams in the meal) following training. If you drink water without eating salty foods during the 2-hour window after training, a large portion (25–50%) of what you drink will be excreted as urine. Here is an interesting side note detailing how much of the following fluids are actually retained in our bodies when we drink after training:

- Caffeinated diet-cola: 50–60%
- Water: 60–70%
- Sports drink: 65–75%

Since muscles are comprised of roughly 60–70% water, it would be most beneficial for you to drink a beverage, such as a sports drink, that will have a higher retention rate to ensure proper re-hydration.

Looking to the Future

A relatively new concept in recovery nutrition that has not received much attention yet is the amount of dietary fat needed for an athlete to recover from exercise. It is possible that the same 130–160 pound athlete we looked at earlier can lose 50–100 grams of intramuscular triglyceride and 50 grams of adipose tissue triglyceride during a hard or long training session. While research doesn't support whether or not this is important in the recovery nutrition performance plan, it is recognized that the increase in body fat oxidation of an endurance athlete is derived almost exclusively from triglyceride fat stored within muscle.

Since this is a fairly new concept in the recovery nutrition plan, there are no specific guidelines for fat consumption post-training. However, it is recommended that you eat 50–100 grams of "healthy" fats (mono- and polyunsaturated) in your normal daily diet (approximately 1 gram of fat per kilogram of body weight).

Recovery Summed Up

The most important nutrients for you to include in your recovery nutrition plan are:

- Water (20–24 ounces per pound of body weight lost)
- High glycemic index carbohydrates such as glucose/dextrose (1.0–1.2 grams per kilogram of body weight)
- Quality protein such as hydrolyzed whey protein and whey protein isolate (6–20 grams)
- Sodium (at least 110–200 milligrams per 8 ounces)
- Glutamine (5–10 grams)

Whether this is accomplished by using a formulated recovery drink with the necessary nutrients or through whole foods is your choice. Remember, your recovery nutrition starts before your training session. Make sure that you are properly fueled before you exercise and replenish lost carbohydrates, water, and electrolytes during exercise.

Last but not least, improvement from intense training happens during sleep, not during your workout. Without proper rest between hard training sessions, your body will not fully recover and improve. If you are not getting enough sleep, it can be a serious detriment to your performance.

SUMMARY

Nutritional supplements as we typically know them include the muscle-building and fat-burning products as well as energy bars, energy gels, sports drinks, and the like. For an endurance athlete, these products aimed at muscle-building and weight loss are simply not important. Your sports drinks, energy bars and gels, recovery drinks, and vitamin and mineral supplements are a focal point of your daily nutrition program and by first understanding what is in each of these products, you can make more educated decisions regarding which ones to try in training and racing.

Remember, nutrition for endurance athletes is a blend of meeting your health and your performance needs. When you choose a product to enhance your performance, keep in mind that your overall health is of great importance also. Do your homework and read the label and ingredients list on all of the nutritional supplements you currently use or are thinking of using before making a decision to use them or not.

6

Special Considerations for the Endurance Athlete

There are a handful of special considerations that I wanted to discuss before the book comes to an end. Many of these issues pertain specifically to you as an endurance athlete and they may also be applicable to you in your quest for better health. Some of the issues I will discuss in this chapter have the potential to negatively impact your performance and health, but with the right amount of knowledge about each, you can prevent most of them from occurring.

I will discuss the following in some detail in this chapter:

- Dehydration
- Heat cramps
- Hyponatremia
- Immune system depression
- The glycemic response

DEHYDRATION

I would be willing to bet that you have experienced some degree of dehydration at some point in your training. Why am I so confident about this? Dehydration is one of the most common ailments among endurance athletes because it doesn't take much at all to become dehydrated. Forget to eat foods that have a high water content or forget to drink enough fluids throughout the day before your workout and most likely, you will experience some level of dehydration during your workout. While you may not think this is an issue, it doesn't take much to affect performance. Before we explore that topic, let me provide a little background about sweating so you have an idea of how dehydration can happen so quickly and be such a serious concern.

Sweating is your body's most effective way of cooling itself; when sweat evaporates from your skin, body heat is reduced. While sweating is important, if you don't replace the fluids you lose through sweat, it can lead to dehydration and heat illness. That's why fluid replacement before, during, and after exercise is so crucial.

When you are training, the heat that is produced by your muscles exceeds the heat released by your body, and your body temperature rises. The increase in your body temperature causes an increase in sweating and blood flow to your skin. The evaporation of sweat removes heat from your skin. Your body can also lose heat through the processes of radiation, conduction, and convection. The four ways that you can lose heat from your body include:

1. Radiation—when heat radiates from the body to cooler objects such as buildings, walls, trees, earth, and the air.
2. Conduction—when heat is transferred from the body by direct physical contact with substances at lower temperature, which happens when you are swimming in cold water.
3. Convection—when heat is transferred by the movement of cool currents of air or water over the body, which happens when you are cycling.

4. Evaporation—when heat is lost when sweat is converted to water vapor, which happens when you are training in a lower-humidity climate.

Our bodies are made up of approximately 55–65% fluid and have 2–4 million sweat glands. The area that has the most sweat glands is the bottom of the feet; the back is the area that has the fewest. Women have more sweat glands than men but men have more active sweat glands and typically have a higher sweat rate. When some of the body's fluid is lost through sweat, it affects the cardiovascular system and the ability to control temperature.

How do you know if you are a heavy sweater? Notice what I call the "soak factor" of your clothing after you finish exercising. If your clothing is dripping wet, then you are a heavy sweater. This can also be measured more precisely in a laboratory setting, but the important thing to remember is that if you are a heavy sweater, you will need more fluids, and possibly sodium, during training to prevent dehydration. More on that later, but let me first explain some of the factors that can influence your sweat rate so you can better control them.

- Environment. No matter where you live, chances are good that you train in at least one warm season. The higher temperatures in warmer seasons can cause you to sweat more quickly and to lose more fluids. Add to that the humidity index and you could be staring dehydration in the eyes. Because humidity affects your body's ability to cool itself, it is harder for sweat to evaporate in hot, humid weather (such as that found in Florida) than in hot, dry weather (such as that found in Colorado). The dryer the environment, the more likely you can become dehydrated in it. Get to know your environment and plan your training and hydration needs accordingly. Remember also that even if it is cold, that doesn't mean that you should drink less. Your body is still sweating and while you may not feel it as much as you would in the heat, you still need to stay hydrated.

- Clothing and equipment. The amount and type of clothing that you wear could contribute to dehydration. By wearing clothing that wicks away sweat and does not hold sweat to your body, you will be able to provide an effective medium of sweat dissipation. Wearing 100% cotton or a lot of equipment that will not allow your body heat to be released as efficiently will increase your chances of becoming dehydrated.

- Fitness and acclimatization. When you increase your fitness level throughout the year, your body becomes more efficient and actually begins to sweat sooner. Some athletes perceive early sweating as a distraction but this distraction is very beneficial because it is a sign that your body has become better at regulating its core temperature to keep you cool. You may see a significant difference in your sweat rate and amount as you progress from your preparation to competition periodization training cycle. You should almost plan on it, especially in your fluid intake needs. In addition, heat will play a big role. As it is usually warmer during the competition cycle, be sure to increase your fluid needs accordingly.

Now that you understand some of the factors that affect how much you can sweat, let's discuss the implications of dehydration. It doesn't matter if you have a high sweat rate or not. Dehydration affects every endurance athlete sometime during their training.

To understand the true effects of dehydration, we must look at it from a physiological perspective. The most serious consequence of exercise-induced dehydration is hyperthermia, which places added stress on the cardiovascular system. Because we are already stressing our cardiovascular systems to some extent during training, this added stress is not beneficial. Dehydration causes fluid to be lost throughout the body. As a result, this increases the concentration and osmolality of dissolved substances and particles in our body's fluids, including the concentration of sodium. These increases in osmolality and in sodium concentration reduce blood flow to the skin and thus decrease the rate of sweating. Definitely not a good thing for an endurance athlete!

Another negative consequence of dehydration-induced hyperthermia is a large decline in cardiac output. Cardiac output is the volume of blood pumped by the heart per minute. A decrease in cardiac output can result in less blood—and therefore less oxygen-being delivered to the working muscles, which means that you cannot train as well. This also reduces the transfer of heat from the body core to the skin, so the body core temperature begins to increase. This is extremely hazardous because we need to remain as cool as possible to continue to train and race, and an increase in the body core temperature can lead to heat exhaustion, heat stroke, and even death in extreme cases.

The primary benefit of sufficient fluid replacement during exercise is that it helps to maintain cardiac output and allows blood flow to the skin to increase to high levels, which will promote heat dissipation from the skin, thereby preventing excessive storage of body heat.

Dehydration can have a negative impact on training and racing with as little as 1% loss of body weight through sweat. If you do the math, this isn't much. If you are a 120-pound endurance athlete, this is only 1.2 pounds that you can lose! If you are training in a warmer environment, you can easily lose this weight in a matter of a training session (and probably much more), and dehydration coupled with warmer temperatures could also put you at risk of developing heat illness. Research has shown that dehydration can happen in as little as 30 minutes in a warmer, humid environment.

Avoiding Dehydration

So what should you do to try to prevent dehydration? Hydrate of course! Drink early, drink often. But be careful what you drink. Water alone is not an effective hydrator because it turns off our thirst response early and turns on our kidneys to get rid of fluids before we have a chance to fully replenish our stores. On average, athletes only replace about 30–60% of their sweat loss by drinking normally, and depending on the thirst response sometimes even less. Sports drinks with adequate sodium will be your best choice for staying hydrated.

Have you ever noticed that after you drink a sports drink, you are still thirsty? Well, this is actually a good thing. A well-formulated sports drink will drive you to drink, which will mean that you will hopefully prevent dehydration. The sodium in sports drinks allows the fluid and carbohydrate to enter your cells, meaning you remain hydrated.

Plus, it can take up to 24 hours to completely re-hydrate if we only drink water. I have yet to meet an endurance athlete who can afford to take 24 hours before filling up their fluid "gas tank" again. And if you are thinking that you will wait until you are thirsty or a bit dehydrated to start drinking, think again. This can cause severe gastrointestinal distress and could lead to stopping during a training session or dropping out of a race. The point is, don't underestimate the power of dehydration. Choose a sports drink that you like, that you will drink, and drink it often before, during, and after training. Refer to Chapter 3, Nutrition Periodization, for the exact quantities of fluids and when you should drink them.

One last note about dehydration: as we age, our perception of thirst actually decreases, so it is important to make a concerted effort to drink often throughout the day as we get older.

HEAT CRAMPS

Not only do you have to worry about dehydration but you also need to be aware of one of the effects of dehydration-heat cramps. Heat cramps are usually caused by salt loss and dehydration. They can occur during prolonged training when there has been profuse and repeated sweating like you would encounter during a longer training session or race. Large losses of fluid and sodium can be factors that can predispose you to heat cramps. Because sodium plays an important role in initiating signals from nerves and actions that lead to movement of the muscles, a sodium deficit could short-circuit the coordination of nerves and muscles. This could result in selected motor nerve endings becoming hyperexcitable and result in spontaneous muscle contractions or cramping.

Sweat and Sodium Losses

In warm to hot conditions, you can lose around 1–2½ liters of sweat per hour (1 liter is equal to approximately 34 ounces). During a longer race or competition, it would not be unheard of for you to lose as much as 10 liters! How much water you lose depends on many factors described previously including temperature, humidity, solar radiation, intensity of exercise, heat acclimatization status, and your fitness level. An increase in any one of these will increase your sweating.

Sweat is mostly comprised of water but also contains the minerals sodium, chloride, potassium, calcium, and magnesium. However, the amounts of potassium, calcium, and magnesium are very low compared to the amounts of sodium and chloride. Also, potassium, calcium, and magnesium are easily replaced by the diet and the muscles tend to stockpile them more than sodium and chloride.

How much sodium can you lose in a training session or race? If you are a well-conditioned athlete who is fully acclimatized to the heat you could have sodium losses of 115–690 milligrams per liter of sweat. If you are not acclimatized to the heat you can have sodium losses of 920–2,300 milligrams per liter of sweat. And as your sweat rates go up, so does your loss of sodium. It is common for a heavy sweater to lose 2,500–5,000 milligrams of sodium per hour in a hot environment. Over an extended training session or race, this could translate into a 15–30% deficit in the total body exchangeable sodium! Note that one teaspoon of salt has 2,400 milligrams of sodium.

In addition to these enormous salt losses, what if you are salt-sensitive or follow a low-salt diet? This makes you more susceptible to heat cramps, especially in hot and humid environments because you are starting with a lower sodium reserve.

Preventing Heat Cramps

Since we know you will lose moderate to large amounts of fluid and sodium during exercise, it only makes sense to replace these during training. Consuming a sports drink that contains 200 milligrams of sodium per 8 ounces is the first step in trying to ward off heat cramps during exercise. However, depending on your sweat rate, sweat sodium concentration, duration, and location of your training and/or race, this may not be nearly enough sodium to prevent cramping.

What can you do to increase the amount of sodium you get? The easiest way is to first concentrate on your regular eating and make sure to follow a diet higher in sodium. In addition, you can add 1/4 teaspoon of salt per 20-ounce bottle of fluid. And finally you can use salt tablets. Be forewarned though that a high amount of sodium delivered all at once into the body, such as in the form of a salt tablet, may shift your water-sodium balance out of whack and predispose you to hypernatremia (a high amount of salt in the blood). If you use salt tablets, choose ones that have minimal salt in them to begin with so you can determine how your body reacts to them. If you will use salt tablets, I recommend starting with ones that have 200 milligrams of sodium or less.

Re-hydrating after Training or Competition

It will be close to impossible for you to keep up with heavy sweat losses during your training or competition. Your goal should be to try to replace the sodium and fluid that you lose as much as possible to prevent a negative impact on your performance. That said, fluid and sodium intake after training or competition is just as important, if not more important, than during the event. The reason is because you will undoubtedly be training again about 12–24 hours afterwards and it is very important that your body is re-hydrated and sodium stores are normal again before beginning another training session, even if it is only a recovery training session.

Re-hydration is a bit tricky because we sometimes don't feel like drinking much after training or a race. You obviously should consume more fluid than what you lost through sweat because some fluid continues to be lost through urine during the re-hydration period. In fact, you should try to replace 150% of your sweat losses. You can do this by drinking 24 ounces for each pound lost.

Here is an example to help you better understand this.

- If you are a 120-pound female endurance athlete and you lost 3 pounds during your training session, then you should begin your re-hydrating by drinking at least 72 ounces of a sports drink (with carbohydrates and sodium) immediately afterwards.
- I know this sounds like a bit much but research has proven this amount to be very effective in re-hydrating the body so that it can recover more quickly.

While specific sodium guidelines do not exist because of the high amount of individuality of sweat rate and sweat sodium concentration, it is important to include some sodium in your re-hydration process because sodium helps to facilitate glucose and water entry into your body's cells. Pure water or a beverage lacking sodium should not be used for re-hydration because your body will not be able to get all of the water inside its cells without sodium and glucose. Most of the water will simply be lost as urine. That means that if you re-hydrate with only water, you will find that you urinate much more because your body is not holding the water for re-hydration. Urinating a lot after your training session or race is not a good thing if you are trying to re-hydrate and recover properly.

Preventing heat cramps begins with replacing fluid and sodium losses during and after training or competition. If you know you are a salty sweater or if you expect to have a higher sweat rate because of the environment or duration of exercise then you should add more sodium to your daily diet and the sports drinks you will use during training or competition.

All this talk about hydration and heat cramps wouldn't be complete without explaining the last big hitter among the three heat- and hydration-related issues that endurance athletes face— hyponatremia.

HYPONATREMIA

Hyponatremia is a disorder in fluid-electrolyte balance that results in an abnormally low plasma sodium concentration. In the 1998 New Zealand Ironman triathlon, 18% of finishers were diagnosed with hyponatremia. This is an alarming number of athletes and this trend is becoming more and more common. Why? Because when you combine a hot environment and a salty sweater with a high sweat rate and improper nutrition, you have a case of hyponatremia just waiting to surface.

The sometimes hot and humid environments that endurance events are held in can greatly affect your ability to finish the race. This type of environmental stress combined with the amount you sweat can spell trouble for you and is certain to result in hyponatremia unless you adopt a sound nutrition plan centered on proper fluid and sodium intake.

Symptoms of Hyponatremia

Some of the symptoms associated with hyponatremia include:

- Gastrointestinal discomfort
- Nausea and vomiting
- Throbbing headache
- Restlessness

- Lethargy
- Confusion
- Respiratory distress
- Seizures
- Brainstem herniation
- Death

The risk of developing complications from hyponatremia depends somewhat on the measured level of plasma sodium in your body.

Here are the physiological ranges of plasma sodium so you have an idea of the numbers that health professionals refer to:

- Normal: 136–142 mmol/L
- Mild hyponatremia: 125–135 mmol/L
- Severe hyponatremia: <125 mmol/L

There have been many studies that have measured plasma sodium concentrations during and after exercise and although the physiological ranges of plasma sodium will provide you an idea of the severity of hyponatremia, the numbers do not always tell the whole story.

For example, athletes have survived hyponatremia when their plasma sodium concentration was in the "severe" category; others have died when their levels were in the "severe" category. If you think that you may be an at-risk athlete, it is important to account for the following variables into your overall nutrition plan:

- Length of training or race—longer races will mean a greater chance of developing hyponatremia.
- Sweat rate—heavy sweaters may be more likely to develop hyponatremia if their fluid consumption is not enough to support their sweat losses.
- Sweat sodium content—salty sweaters may be more likely to develop hyponatremia than non-salty sweaters if their sodium intake is not high enough to support their sodium losses.

By knowing these three things ahead of time and with some proper planning before your training session or race, you can reduce your risk of developing hyponatremia. Hyponatremia cannot be prevented during exercise but the risk can be reduced by proper planning.

Causes of Hyponatremia

What causes hyponatremia? There are many factors that can cause hyponatremia but the most common is excessive fluid intake. With excessive water intake, there is an increased risk of developing hyponatremia because your body's sodium levels decrease. In addition, sodium loss from sweat is increased, which makes it even easier to dilute your body's sodium content.

While some researchers believe hyponatremia is associated with fluid overload, others believe it is associated with dehydration. What is important to realize is if you are training or competing in an event in which you will have prolonged sweating, this may predispose you to hyponatremia. The balance of fluid intake and sodium intake and the timing of fluid intake become of utmost importance, which is one thing many researchers can agree upon.

Prevention of Hyponatremia

So now you know what hyponatremia is and the main cause of it, but what you really want to know is how to prevent it. Prevention of hyponatremia must include a combination of knowing if you are an at-risk athlete and knowing how to properly plan to try to prevent hyponatremia.

Identification of your at-risk status should be your first step. Determine your sweat rate and sweat sodium content. If you want accuracy, the best place to have these measured is in a human performance laboratory that offers this testing. If you don't have access to this, you can take a more simple, yet not as quantitative, approach. You will know during your training if you have a high sweat rate because your clothes will be drenched with sweat on a consistent basis by the time you finish a workout. And if your clothes have a white residue on them after every training session, then you can probably conclude that you are somewhat of a salty sweater. Again, this at-home assessment method will not provide you exact numbers, but it will help you determine if you are an at-risk athlete.

Once you identify whether you are at risk or not, your next step is to educate and protect yourself. If you are at risk, adopt the following strategies in your nutrition plan:

- Maintain a diet that has enough sodium (as long as you have no pre-existing medical conditions that would make salt consumption detrimental). You probably already consume more than the recommended daily amount of sodium, 2,400 milligrams, anyway. Most people do because of the food selection in our society and the abundance of sodium in most foods.

- Consume sodium during exercise. Sports drinks, pretzels, and salt tablets or powders work; however, use caution when using salt tablets or powder. As I described previously, interdepartmental fluid shifts (when the sodium concentration inside our bodies increases or decreases due to more or less water intake) can be seen when too much sodium is introduced into the body without adequate fluid. Hypernatremia can develop as a result of harboring too much sodium without enough fluid. Then you have a whole other issue to worry about!

- Drink accordingly based on sweat rate. If you do not know your sweat rate, then you should follow the general recommendations covered in Chapter 3. Drink 7–10 ounces of a sports drink containing sodium every 15–20 minutes then customize consumption based on your body, training environment, and duration of exercise.

- Avoid overdrinking. I cannot emphasize this point more strongly. You have read what drinking too much water can do to you in the first two sections of this chapter. Stick to your fluid and sodium intake plan that you determine beforehand. I have seen too many athletes deviate from their plan during a race and take an extra cup or two of water at each aid station. They have paid dearly for it later in the race or at the end of the race with IV "cocktails" hooked up to them. Make a plan and stick with it.

- Limit pre-hydration. This can lower your blood sodium before the event begins and leave you behind in your sodium intake plan. Follow the general guidelines presented in Chapter 3 of drinking 17–20 ounces of a sports drink containing sodium 2 hours before exercise and 7–10 ounces 10–20 minutes before the start of exercise.

- Don't overdrink after training or competition. Weight loss of 1–2 pounds during an exercise bout can indicate dehydration. If you are an at-risk athlete, you should get into the habit of weighing yourself before and after exercise to determine your exact fluid needs afterwards. Remember, drink 20–24 ounces of sports drink for every pound that you lose during an event.

Knowing the risks and symptoms of hyponatremia is important any time of the year that you are training. Knowing your individual sweat rate and sweat sodium concentration is helpful so you can plan your fluid and sodium needs. However, if you can't have these measured, simply follow the fluid and sodium guidelines presented earlier in this book and fine-tune them to your body as you find necessary. Sports drinks should always be favored over water during exercise so you make sure you consume the necessary fluid, carbohydrates, and sodium.

IMMUNE SYSTEM DEPRESSION

How many times a year do you get sick? I am sure you continually wonder if your latest ailment is training-related or if you just caught the illness from a friend or family member. Well, there is some very good research that confirms that endurance training may be associated with an increased risk of illness. While this surely isn't always the case, it is something to be extremely aware of and take extra time to plan to keep your immune system healthy.

Regular, moderate exercise is great for keeping you in good health, but more intense workouts, such as intervals or hill repeats, may actually suppress the immune system and increase your chances of getting sick. The increased susceptibility for illness after exercise is thought to be related to the increase in stress hormones during and after exercise. This can last between 3 and 72 hours and during this time viruses and bacteria can exert their negative effects on your body.

Cortisol

Let's discuss one of the main culprits in the stress hormone family. Cortisol is a hormone controlled by the adrenal cortex (our body's factory for producing steroid hormones) and is known to be the regulator of the immune system. Its primary functions are to increase protein breakdown in our muscles, inhibit the uptake of glucose into our body's cells, and increase the breakdown of fats. Cortisol levels can have a negative impact on many different areas in our body including sleep, mood, bone health, ligament health, cardiovascular health, and athletic performance.

So, what does this mean for you, the endurance athlete? High levels of cortisol may result when you don't pay close attention to your daily nutrition. A chronically elevated amount of cortisol causes fat, protein, and carbohydrates to be mobilized quickly While this is happening, two other hormones, testosterone and DHEA (dehydroepiaandrosterone), decrease. Your body enters a constant state of muscle breakdown and suppressed immune function. It's a vicious cycle that repeats itself over and over when you don't follow a sound eating program. More about that later, but let me discuss what this can do to your performance.

Chronically high levels of cortisol suppress the immune system and decrease your level of testosterone. In addition, high cortisol levels can put you at greater risk for developing upper respiratory-tract infections (often referred to as URTIs). This isn't rocket science. The more you are sick, the less you get to exercise to improve health and performance. Some researchers have shown that using the ratio of anabolic to catabolic steroids (i.e., the ratio of testosterone to cortisol) can provide results that can help to assess an athlete's training state. A ratio that favors increased cortisol can indicate overtraining.

If you train in a carbohydrate-depleted state (i.e., follow a daily low-carbohydrate diet), you could experience a greater amount of cortisol in your body. Unfortunately, high intensity and long duration training both increase cortisol levels. If you are trying to improve your speed or are training for an event lasting longer than 3–4 hours, chances are that you have a high amount of cortisol in your body. This remains elevated for about 2 hours after you finish training, which means, as I keep saying, your daily nutrition plan is of utmost importance.

But how do you actually know if your cortisol levels are high? It just so happens that there are a few easy-to-recognize symptoms that lead you to the answer without having your cortisol levels measured. Symptoms of high cortisol levels include mood swings, lack of motivation to train, and loss of muscle and appetite. I keep mentioning the power of nutrition to help control cortisol levels. Regulating and controlling cortisol levels doesn't begin during or after training. It begins in your daily eating program. As I stated before, carbohydrates can help decrease the cortisol response, so if you follow a daily eating program that has moderate to high amounts of carbohydrates, you will be taking the first step in cortisol control. Going into a workout without adequate carbohydrate stores will set you up for improper recovery as well as for the negative impact that high cortisol levels have following exercise, which I have already discussed. In addition, research has shown that eating a higher-carbohydrate meal prior to your training and during training will also help control the cortisol increase in your body. Some good research has also demonstrated that the addition of glutamine and branched-chain amino acids during your post-exercise nutrition plan can also help to modulate cortisol release.

So there you have it. Follow a moderate- to high-carbohydrate diet, eat a higher-carbohydrate meal before training, eat carbohydrates during training and follow the recommended nutrition recovery principles covered in Chapter 3, possibly adding glutamine and branched-chain amino acids to it, and you will be able to control your cortisol levels following training and prevent any of the negative side effects the hormone can elicit in your body. You can choose solid food to get these nutrients or a recovery-type beverage. The choice is up to you and really depends on what you can eat or drink after a training session or race. Customize your post-recovery nutrition plan to your specific needs and wants.

Glycemic Response

The glycemic response (GR) of a food is a measure of that food's ability to raise blood glucose (blood sugar). The two key players in determining GR are glycemic index (GI) and glycemic load (GL). Many endurance athletes are adopting the use of GI but, unfortunately, the GL is not often being used in conjunction with it; therefore, the athlete is plagued with misinformation and is using only one-half of the puzzle. Let me discuss this in more detail so you can understand what using the overall glycemic response truly means.

Glycemic Index

The Glycemic Index has existed for a while but it has been gaining more popularity recently due to its featured role in new "fad" diets. Simply put, GI is a standard measure of how quickly 50 grams of a particular food's carbohydrates are converted to sugar and thus affect our blood sugar over a 2-hour period. The GI has existed for decades and has been used by registered dietitians specifically in their counseling with individuals with diabetes.

As you may remember from Chapter 2, simple carbohydrates are those with only one or two sugar units in a chain while complex carbohydrates are those with hundreds to thousands of these units in a single chain. In the past, simple carbohydrates were classified as having a high GI, that is, causing a quick rise and fall in blood sugar, and complex carbohydrates were classified as providing sustained energy with a more gentle rise in blood sugar. When it came to the GI, simple carbohydrates were classified as "bad" and complex carbohydrates as "good".

While this may seem fairly logical, recent data indicates that this concept is out of date. Non-refined, or wholesome, carbohydrates are always preferred because they provide important nutrients whereas refined carbohydrates do not and therefore should be limited in your diet. However, many athletes correlate wholesome with complex and simple with refined, and that is simply not the case. For example, fruit is considered a simple carbohydrate but these carbohydrates are unrefined and fruit is very nutrient-dense, meaning it has many vitamins and minerals and a good amount of fiber. It has been shown that each food produces its own blood sugar profile and there is not a strong correlation to whether or not it contains simple or complex carbohydrates. Some complex carbohydrates can be digested, absorbed, and utilized as quickly as simple sugars, meaning that they have similar glycemic responses.

The following is a short list of factors that can affect the GI of foods:

- Biochemical structure of the carbohydrate
- Absorption process
- Size of meal
- Degree of processing
- Contents and timing of previous meal

- Fat, fiber, and protein content
- Ripeness

You can see that the GI of a carbohydrate is dependent upon many factors other than just the complexity of the carbohydrate. It is impossible to classify a food as "healthy" or "unhealthy" simply based on its complex or simple chemical structure or based solely on its GI. GI tells you how fast a carbohydrate will increase your blood sugar levels but it doesn't tell you how much of that carbohydrate is in a serving of that food. This is where glycemic load comes into play. Both the GI and GL are needed to truly determine what glycemic response that food will have on your body. I don't mean to be confusing; you can and will see that using this process for daily food selection will become quite overwhelming. I will provide my recommendations on how to use this information later, but first, let's learn about glycemic load so you understand all of the pieces of the puzzle.

Glycemic Load

Glycemic load is the numerical value of the glycemic index divided by 100 and multiplied by the food's available carbohydrate content (in grams). GL takes the glycemic index into account, but is based on how much carbohydrate is in the food or drink tested. The glycemic load is numerically lower than the glycemic index of a food or drink.

Here is an example.

- Watermelon has a GI of 72. A recommended serving of 1/2 cup is 4 ounces or 120 grams of watermelon. This serving has 6 grams of carbohydrates.
- To calculate the GL, divide the GI by 100 and multiply by carbohydrate content in grams:

$$(72/100) \times 6 = 4.32, \text{ or 4 when we round}$$

In this example, a high-GI food becomes a low-GL food. So, based on the serving size and quantity of watermelon eaten, it will have a better GR and therefore result in a lower rise in blood sugar than its GI indicates. Keep in mind though that as you increase the serving size eaten, you increase the amount of carbohydrates eaten, which will in turn increase the GR of the food.

In many cases, GL is not based on a typical amount of food eaten, so GL does not provide realistic information, unless the food is weighed prior to consuming it. I am certainly not suggesting that you weigh all of your food before eating it. That is simply not convenient or necessary. The important take-home lesson about GL is that it provides an understanding of the relationship between a specific amount of food and its biochemical response.

Let's look at another example. The GI of ice cream is 37 and the GL is 4, based on consumption of 50 grams of ice cream. Sixty-five grams of ice cream equals 1/2 cup, so 50 grams of ice cream is less than 1/2 cup. Realistically, who eats less than 1/2 cup of ice cream at a time? As the serving size increases, so does the GR.

Table 6.1 lists the ranges that classify food by their respective GI and GL values.

Glycemic index is most useful when deciding which high-carbohydrate foods to eat and when to eat them before, during, and after training. It is generally advised to consume a moderate-GI meal before training, high-GI foods during training, and high-GI foods immediately after training, but this general rule is based only on the science of nutrition. The other half of the equation is the art; you must take the recommendations that science has provided and customize them to your body and its specific needs and

Table 6.1
GI and GL Classifications

Value	Glycemic Index (GI)	Glycemic Load (GL)
High	≥ 70	20
Medium	56–69	11–19
Low	≤ 55	≤ 10

wants. In this confusing yet informative section about glycemic response, I hope I have accomplished three things:

1. Provided you enough information for you to consider factoring in the concept of glycemic response as you design your personal nutrition plan.
2. Proved to you that using GI or GL by itself is not useful and that the two concepts must be considered together.
3. Illustrated that while the GR of foods is important, it is not mandatory that you follow it with all of your meals all of the time. Focusing on the basic nutrition recommendations of eating fruits and vegetables, whole grains, lean meats, and lower-fat foods with a lot of variety and of reducing the amount of refined foods should always be your focus. Food is fun and is an important part of our lives. Don't get caught up in numbers all of the time and allow the enjoyment of eating slip to your waist side.

SUMMARY

You know better than anyone whether or not a food or drink will be right for you at a specific time. Don't adopt a nutrition plan just because it works for your friend, family member, or training partner, and please don't choose a product because a professional sports figure endorses it. Individualize your nutrition to your body and your training to elicit the most positive health and performance benefits possible.

Index

Alanine 25
Alcohol 105, 106
Amine group 23
Amino acids 23, 24
  branched-chain 126
  essential 24–25
  nonessential 25
  oxidation 21
Arginine 25
Asparagine 25
Aspartic acid 25
Athletic Banned Substances Screened
  Products Program 127

Base
  cycle. *See* Mesocycle, preparation.
  training 7
Beta-carotene 52
Beta-hydroxy-beta-methylbutyrate
  127
Biotin 37

Body Media 112
Brown rice syrup 141
Build cycle. *See* Mesocycle,
  competition.
Build-to-recover model 13

Caffeine 139
Calcium 134
Cancer 71
Carbohydrates 16, 18–22, 50, 58,
  64–65, 67, 68, 69, 74, 76, 79, 80,
  81, 96, 105, 106, 130, 134, 143,
  146, 163, 164, 165, 166, 167, 168
  complex 19
  and the endurance athlete 20–22
  loading 82–87, 89
  simple 18–19
  sources of 19–20
Cardiac output 153
Cardiovascular disease 28, 29, 30, 41,
  71

Carnitine 126
Conduction 150
Conjugated linoleic acid 126
Constipation 71
ConsumerLabs.com 127, 139
Convection 150
Cortisol 163–165
Cramps, heat 149, 154–158
Cravings 54
Creatine 126
Cysteine 25

Dehydration 137, 149, 150–154, 160
Dextrose 132, 133
Dietary Supplements Health and Education Act 124
Dietitian, registered, 114, 115
Diets, fad 109–111
Digestion 17
Disaccharides 19
Diuretic 139
Doping 125

Electrolytes 131, 144–145
Endurance training, cornerstones of 47, 48
Energy
  bars 72, 77, 87, 137–140
  gels 72, 77, 87, 140–142
Ergogenic 128
Exercise expenditure 107–108
Evaporation 151

Fat 16, 26–32, 50, 55, 62, 65, 74, 79, 84, 86, 96, 105, 106, 145–146
  poly/monounsaturated vs. saturated/trans 52–53
  sources of 31–32
  types of 28–31
Fatty acids
  essential 29–31

omega-3 29–31
omega-6 29–31
Fiber 16, 41–43, 44, 71, 88, 140
  types of 42–43
Folic acid 37
Food and Drug Administration 127, 129
Food diary 53–54
Fractionated palm kernel oil 137–138
Fructose 19, 130, 132, 133, 134, 141

Galactose 19, 132, 133, 134
Gastrointestinal distress 16
Glucose 18, 19, 130, 132, 133, 141, 143
  polymers 132, 133
Glutamic acid 25
Glutamine 25, 126, 144, 146
Glycemic
  response 149, 165–169
  index value 133, 165–167, 168, 169
  load 167–169
Glycerin 138–139
Glycine 25
Glycogen 18
  muscle 143–144
Green tea extract 134, 139–140
Group program 117
Guarana 126

HealthTech, Inc. 112
Heat
  exhaustion 153
  stroke 153
Herbal extracts 127
High blood pressure 77
Hill repeats 8
Histidine 24
Honey 141
Hormones, stress 163
Hydration 34, 38, 62–63, 66–68,

74–75, 80, 81, 82, 87, 90, 96, 97,
  144–145, 151, 153–154, 156–158,
  161, 162
Hypernatremia 156
Hyperthermia 152, 153
Hyponatremia 90, 93, 131, 149,
  158–162

Illness 162–164
Immune system depression 149,
  162–165
Injury 10
Insulin 134, 135, 143
Intensity cycle. *See* Mesocycle, compe-
  tition.
International Olympic Committee
  125, 126
Iron 53
Ironman 90–95
Isoleucine 24

Korr 112

Lactate threshold 8
Lactose 19
Leucine 24
Lifestyle change 102
Lipoprotein
  high-density 29
  low-density 29
Log
  food 114–115
  physical activity 115–116
Long slow distance (LSD) training 7
Lysine 24

Macrocycle 6
  guidelines 51–57
Macronutrient needs 58–66, 74–75,
  79–80, 96–97
  and fluid timing 66–69, 75–76,

80–82, 97–98
  and weight 59–61
Magnesium 134
Maltodextrin 132, 133
Maltose 19
Mesocycle 6
  competition 8, 9, 73–95
    pre-race cycle 74–78
      daily nutrition needs 74–75
      eating guidelines 72–78
      macronutrient and fluid timing
        75–76
    race cycle 78–95
      carbohydrate loading 82–87
      daily nutrition needs 79–80
      eating guidelines 87–90
      macronutrient and fluid timing
        80–82
  preparation 7, 9, 57–73
    daily nutrition needs 63–66
    macronutrient and fluid timing
      66–69
    recovery nutrition for 69–70
  transition 95–99, 103, 104, 105
    daily nutrition needs 96–97
    eating guidelines 98–99
    macronutrient and fluid timing
      97–98
Methionine 24
Microcycles 6–7
Minerals 16, 38–41, 126
  calcium 39
  chromium 40
  copper 40
  fluoride 40
  iodine 40
  iron 39
  magnesium 39
  manganese 40
  phosphorus 41
  potassium 39

selenium 40
sodium 39
zinc 40
Monosaccharides 19
Multivitamin 53

Nandrolone 125
National Nutritional Foods Association 127
New Leaf 112
Niacin 37
NSF International 127
Nutrients 15–45
    essential 16
Nutrition periodization 47–100
    components of 6
    definition of 5
    history of 6
    specifics of 50–51

Occupational/ lifestyle expenditure 107
Off season 9
Oligosaccharides 19
Osmolality 131
Overload 10
Overreaching 10, 11
Overtraining 10–12
    definition of 11
    signs of 11–12

Pantothenic acid 37
Periodization. *See* Nutrition periodization.
Personal Energy Balance Equation (PEBE) 105–108, 113, 114, 116, 117
Phenylalanine 24
Phospholipids 26
Phytochemicals 71
Pilates 7

Plyometrics 8
Polyols 138
Polysaccharides 19
Pregnancy 35, 36
Preparation cycle 103, 104
Pre-race cycle. *See* Mesocycle, competition, pre-race.
Prohormones 125
Proline 25
Protein 16, 22–26, 50, 56–57, 58, 62, 65, 70, 74, 79, 84, 86, 96, 105, 134–135, 143, 144, 146
    hydrolyzed whey 144
    powders 127
    serving sizes of 25–26
    sources of 25
    in sports drinks 134–137
    types of 24–25
Pyruvate 127

Race cycle. *See* Mesocycle, competition, race.
Radiation 150
Recovery 10, 12–13
    cycle. *See* Mesocycle, transition.
    drinks 142–146
Resting metabolic rate (RMR) 108, 109, 110, 111, 113, 114, 116–117
    measuring 111–113
Retinol 36
Rheumatoid arthritis 30
Riboflavin 36
Ribose 126

Salt tablets 77, 88, 156, 161
Serine 25
Sleep 146
Snacking 77
Sodium 77, 87, 88, 131, 146, 152, 153, 155–158, 161
Special considerations 149–169

Spices 89
Sports drinks 66, 67–68, 72, 75, 77,
    81, 87, 98, 130–137, 154, 156,
    157, 161
  protein in 134–137
  sugars in 131–134
Sport-specific drills 9
Step counter 116
Steroids 126
Stroke 41
Sucrose 19, 130, 132, 133
Sugar 130, 131–134
  alcohol 138
  in sports drinks 131–134
Supplements, nutritional 55, 123–147
  contamination 125–127
  energy bars 137–140
  energy gels 140–142
  recovery 142–146
  sports drinks 130–137
Sweating 150–153, 155, 159, 160,
    161

Testosterone 125
Thermic effect of food 106–107
Thermogenesis 107, 139
Thiamin 36
Thirst 33
Threonine 24
Training
  physiological 47, 48
  psychological 47, 48
  strength 8
  year 5, 6
Transition cycle. *See* Mesocycle, tran-
    sition.
Tribulus terrestris 126
Triglycerides 26
Tryptophan 25
Tyrosine 25

United States Pharmacopoeia 129

Valine 25
Vegan 57
Vegetarian 36
Vitamins 126, 134
  A (retinal) 36
  B_1 (thiamin) 36
  B_2 (riboflavin) 36
  B_3 (niacin) 37
  B_6 37
  B_{12} 37
  Biotin 37
  C 38, 52
  D 38
  E 38, 52
  Folic acid 37
  K 38
  Pantothenic acid 37
VO_2 max 8

Water 16, 32–34, 146, 153, 154, 157,
    160, 161
  body 144–145
Weight
  gain 82, 95–96
  loss 58, 73
    basics of 105–109
    fad diets 109–111
    how to achieve 113–122
    and resting metabolic rate
      111–113
    timing 102–105
  management 101–122
Window of opportunity
    142–143

Yoga 7

Zinc 52, 126

Base

	CHO (g/kg)	PRO (g/kg)
	5-7 g/kg mod-low	1.2 g 1.7
	7-12 g mod-high	

Comp

Pre Race	7-13 g	1.4 - 2.0 g
RACE	same	

During Exercise

Base

	CHO	PRO
During	30-60 g / HR	X
After: 30 min	1-1.2 g/kg	6-20 g
2 HR	1-1.2 g/kg	X
Pre-Race	same	
Race		

wt = 130 lb = 59 kg

BMR = 1300 (Harris-Benedict)

11.9 cal/min — bike
~ run

1300 × 1.6 = 2,000 cal/d